Nathalie Marie-Claire grew up in a French-speaking family in Montreal. She has a natural affinity for cultivating meaningful relationships and reflecting thoughtfully on her personal experiences and those of others. Her incessant curiosity about all things and full-hearted engagement in the difficulties and joys of life have led her to write her first book, *For ALL It's Worth, Because You Matter.* This book reveals wisdom from unusual sources, reflections from deeply transformative personal stories and insightful travel tales. Her intention is to share what she has received with those who seek healing and growth in their own lives. Nathalie now lives in London.

For my daughter,
my eternal sunshine

Nathalie Marie-Claire

FOR ALL IT'S WORTH, BECAUSE YOU MATTER

AUSTIN MACAULEY PUBLISHERS™

LONDON • CAMBRIDGE • NEW YORK • SHARJAH

A CIP catalogue record for this title is available from the British Library.

ISBN 9781398473799 (Paperback)
ISBN 9781398473805 (Hardback)
ISBN 9781398473829 (ePub e-book)
ISBN 9781398473812 (Audiobook)

www.austinmacauley.com

First Published 2023
Austin Macauley Publishers Ltd®
1 Canada Square
Canary Wharf
London
E14 5AA

Acknowledgements

This first book writing journey has been an exploration into the challenges and beauty of life. In always keeping in mind the objective of helping at least one reader, it motivated me to bring it to life. The support and encouragement of some dear friends have kept me going, and I would like to thank them. In particular, I'd like to thank Sara for believing in me, for the time she graciously took to go over my manuscript, for her insightful observations and suggestions, for her honest comments prompting me to challenge my thinking and writing and for her loving prayers.

I would also like to thank – with all my heart – my daughter, who loves me through my flaws, who is my best friend and travel partner, whose support I couldn't do without and whose strength of character inspires me always. My mother who is the embodiment of care and thoughtfulness. Her actions have taught me so much and shaped a big part of who I am today. My father, who is a role model for discipline, perseverance and whose loving presence can be felt from miles away. His calmness and objectivity amidst hardships is a trait I have come to appreciate gradually in my adulthood. My sister, whose unfailing love and courage are a true blessing to me and everyone around her. My nephew, whose innate artistic talents have brought life to the contents of this book through beautiful illustrations. My godson, whose unwavering loyalty and pure love inspire me. Denis, my brother in heart and laughter. Graham, for his unwavering support and for all the amazing things and precious moments we have shared together. His passion for people and for what he engages in, and builds, have also inspired me to make this project come to light.

My sincere thanks to Troels, who has wholeheartedly contributed to shining a personal light on the subject of discipline and freedom. His journey, insights and experience are a great source of inspiration. To Gunnar, whose high standards of teaching and constant aim for excellence have taught me way beyond the dance floor. For his genuineness, dedication and patience. For making my dream come true and for the good laughs. To Marika, for being a glowing example of what embracing one's uniqueness is all about and for encouraging me to explore the freedom to express myself. To my long-time friends Jackie and Catherine for their unfailing presence and treasured friendship. To Salma; little did she know that what she said to me over tea at her house in D.C. almost a decade ago would have been more than just a spark that illuminated this first writing journey, "Everyone has a story to tell. Everyone's story is important." To Edson, for his listening ear and enthusiasm for all I embark on. To Jamie, for the slice of time filled with solace. To Paul, whose exemplary leadership skills and life wisdom elevate my thinking and for our memorable Library Bar chats.

To Craig, for the beautiful cover design and the love it expresses.

To Austin Macauley Publishers for the opportunity to make this book a reality.

Table of Contents

Preface   11

Chapter 1: Discipline   16

An Unexpected Answer

Chapter 2: Matterness and Gentleness   32

Chapter 3: One   41

*The Intrinsic Value of One Lies in Its
Infinite Magnitude*

Chapter 4: Full Presence   53

Superman and the Marshmallow

Chapter 5: Preparedness and Intuition   66

Where Inner Calm Meets the Target

Chapter 6: Forgiveness   76

A Story with Wings

Chapter 7: Deep Minding   87

There Is No Secret

Chapter 8: The Power of Prayer   102

Even If You Don't Know How to Pray

Chapter 9: Your Body and Its Temple   **114**

Chapter 10: The Theory of Everything   **129**

   In Search of Equanimity

Chapter 11: Reminders and Compass-Setters   **145**

Preface

For ALL It's Worth, Because You Matter

Here I am, in my early fifties, going through a divorce. At best an unfamiliar place, taking solace in life's blessings and ever-changing nature. All of a sudden, I have to face this high-definition screen with the whole of my life defiling in front of my eyes. Revisiting it all, the highs and lows, everything. The joys and the torments. The blessings and the longings. How am I now going to keep my life script running? Many characters have changed and I am forced to change.

I decided to delve into books of wisdom and countless hours of podcasts. Jotting down pages of notes, tirelessly reflecting, searching for signs, digging deep in my heart, only to come back to square one. Something was missing.

So, on a mission I was. A quest for an answer, a revelation, which took me all the way to Japan. Only in stillness and peace does anything become clear. This clarity expressed itself through experiencing Japan's mystical calmness. Witnessing all of its beauty and engaging in meaningful encounters paved the way to reshaping my thoughts and life. It turned out that not only would there be a revelation but many answers.

An acquaintance I met during my trip had posted an article on Facebook which made an impression on me. I would even go further, saying it was a sign that I needed to take action. The article he'd shared examined how society is spending more time consuming than creating.

I am therefore devoting myself to bringing you lessons to ponder and stories to inspire. Stories of healing and discovery, inviting you to continue exploring ways to experience harmony in your life and spread it around you.

This creative endeavour was preceded by doubts, residing in my heart for months. Was there even a need for yet another book on personal growth? It's all been said, right? I have never written a book before. My experiences don't even come close to the extreme hardship endured by so many. What more can be squeezed out of healing, forgiveness, awareness, life lessons and self-mastery? Besides, I am not an expert on any of these matters.

Then I thought, that's precisely why I need to write. I remembered a famous quote by Confucius: "Life is really simple, but we insist on making it complicated." My approach to writing is to convey meaningfulness with simplicity.

I do not have it all figured out. There are still days where darkness creeps into the depth of my mind and soul but along the way I found some valuable keys worth using and keeping safe. Some opened doors to seeing the many things I questioned in a different light. Others were keys to finding ways towards harmony.

Regardless of how your life is unfolding, I invite you to follow me on a voyage where my humble thoughts and reflections will help guide you on your own path towards finding calm, freedom, healing and balance in your life. It's about reshaping our thinking, in simple ways, and embracing discipline and gentleness. It's about adopting more constructive and beneficial ways to go about life, and giving you a different appreciation for the marvellous ways in which it manifests its love for you. It's also about giving you the freedom to ponder the ideas I approach throughout. Sharing empowers us both, the giver and the receiver. In all transparency, I am still struggling at times but I know I have keys to help me open and close doors. In sharing them with you, I hope that they will also empower you.

Just before starting this writing journey, I would have titled this book, *For All It's Worth*. But that implies an uncertainty about its significance or usefulness. Today, I'm proud to write '**ALL**' in bold and capital letters. *For **ALL** It's Worth*. All of the incalculable grace we're given and all of the wise lessons that help us transform our lives. All of the challenges we endure and overcome, and all the love we can spread around us.

Through the lenses of God's grace, of my daughter's love, resilience and grit, and her pug's affection, my life's purpose became very clear: To care and to love.

This book is a vehicle to drive this purpose forward and encourage you to join me along the way. I believe that even though we might not know one another, as you read along, I will somehow learn from your stories, too.

There will be books written until the end of time so I chose to go ahead and make mine part of life's library. I thank you for making it part of yours, too.

With love and tenderness,
Nathalie M.C.

All proceeds from this book will be donated to the organisations featured in some of the stories.

OM
KI LI
KA KU
SO WA
KA

Chapter 1
Discipline
An Unexpected Answer

Everyone can adopt a discipline to foster freedom in their life. To transform their life. Discipline is freeing.

The surprising answer was revealed at the culmination of a long walk uphill, braving a hoard of tourists along the way.

No trip to Japan is complete without visiting the Fushimi Inari Shrine just south of Kyoto. Its thousands of vermilion torii gates straddle a network of trails which lead into the wooded forest of the sacred Mount Inari. Fushimi Inari is the most important of several thousands of shrines dedicated to Inari, Shinto god of rice and prosperity. Foxes are thought to be Inari's messengers or guardians, hence the abundance of fox statues adorning the shrine grounds. Fushimi Inari has ancient origins, predating the capital's move to Kyoto in 794.

Going through the first row of torii is jaw-dropping, almost surreal. It's like entering a massive, mysterious and winding bright red tunnel, which seems unending. Thousands upon thousands of magnificent torii gates, donated by corporations and wealthy individuals, arch over the main pathway. Every donor's name is aesthetically inscribed on the back of each gate in shiny black ink. The custom of donating a torii dates back to the Edo period and symbolises hope of receiving good fortune or gratitude for success or a granted wish.

After just under one hour's ascent, my guide and I reached the Yotsutsuji intersection roughly halfway up the mountain, offering stunning views over Kyoto. Most hikers only venture up to that point, as the gate density further decreases, but we carried on and headed to our destination, leaving us to silently connect with nature and with one another.

Beyond wanting to witness the shrine's magnitude and sacredness, I was there for another reason. I was about to immerse myself into another world. The luscious forest which was gradually unfolding around us was about to reveal its secrets.

As I was preparing my trip, a search for spending time in nature with a monk had led me to Kuniatsu, a Buddhist monk offering guided meditation and forest bathing tours. I had heard so much about forest bathing that I longed to experience it in its fullness.

We climbed stoned stairs, followed adjacent paths dotted with smaller shrines enveloped in the gentle smoke of slow burning incense. I was intrigued by the array of seemingly odd offerings that lay at the fox statues' feet: coins, sake bottles, and grains of rice. Questions raced through my head. What were the mysterious powers of the Shinto gods? How did devotees experience them through their faith? As a Christian, I relate to the human nature of one God. Still so much to learn…

Passing gentle flowing streams, we moved through deep shades of green and brown. The air was damp, delightfully cool and the woods' fragrance was intensifying. The last trail split into a circular route to the summit. Steps were uneven and broken. The journey became more arduous as the climb was steep. Kuniatsu was pacing himself, welcoming my string of questions while resting his legs and sharing his knowledge about the shrine and Shinto rituals. Most fascinating.

At one point, he veered off the path and lead me into the forest towards a small, unmarked monastery. He had built up my expectations telling me that if we were lucky, the monks would have left (not sure where to, nor why, but I thought it was not the time to ask!) and we would be able to do our meditation sitting on the wooden porch overlooking the forest. I was excited yet nervous. The art of meditation has clearly been escaping me for years despite my best of intentions. I feel like I've pretty much downloaded all of the mediation apps out there! Nevertheless, their soothing narrative voices bring me slivers of calmness for a few minutes every day.

Back to the forest…

The announcement came: "It's clear, the monks have left, we have it all to ourselves!" Second lucky moment of the day. Kuniatsu told me earlier that a few other people had also signed up to join his tour but cancelled. Regardless, he was truly happy to honour his commitment despite the fact that I was the only person who showed up.

After disappearing momentarily, he came back dressed in loose brown cotton trousers with a kimono-style top and invited me to sit crossed-legged on the porch as he stood on the ground, facing me. Like a tree deeply rooted and connected with Mother Earth. He was about to guide me in a meditation and chanting practice. I was going to chant, me? I can barely concentrate for a few minutes at a time. Plus, I found the chanting in the very few yoga classes I attended years ago rather peculiar, edging on weird. Firstly though, I was dying to ask about the essence of forest bathing. What made it different from a therapeutic walk in the woods? What was the science behind it? He explained that beyond releasing oxygen, trees exchange particles, invisible to the human eye, interacting with us on an energetic level. Those particles interconnect, freely flowing amongst trees, plants, and soil, and shower us with positive energy. They gently touch us, we inhale them, they heal us. They purify our body and soul.

On a scientific level, here is what is said about forest bathing:

From 2004 to 2012, Japanese officials spent about four million dollars studying the physiological and psychological effects of forest bathing, designating 48 therapy trails based on the results. Qing Li, a professor at Nippon Medical School in Tokyo, measured the activity of human natural killer (NK) cells in the immune system before and after exposure to the woods. These cells provide rapid responses to viral infected cells, to tumour formation, and are associated with immune system health and cancer prevention. In a 2009 study, Li's subjects showed significant increases in NK cell activity in the week after a forest visit, and positive effects lasted a month following each weekend in the woods.

This is due to various essential oils, generally called phytoncide, found in wood, plants, and some fruit and vegetables, which trees emit to protect themselves from germs and insects. Forest air doesn't just feel fresher and better; inhaling phytoncide seems to actually improve immune system function.

19

ref. for the two paragraphs above:
https://qz.com/804022/health-benefits-japanese-forest-
bathing/

The breathing and counting meditation took me to a serene place and he made me feel at ease as he too closed his eyes. Thoughts were passing through my mind though, carried by the mysteries of the whole unseen universe. Particles flying around me, holding their own secrets.

Following our meditation, he handed me a little piece of cardboard on which he had written a chanting mantra. It went like this: "OM, KILI, KAKU, SOWA, KA." I was to initially repeat it after him, eyes closed, and as he'd progressively increase the speed, we'd have to chant in synchrony with each other. I could feel my body starting to sweat… I can barely recall the first three digits of a phone number when needed!

Clearly noticing my uneasiness, he paused to teach me the basics about chanting and described how the combination of sound, breath and rhythm moves energy throughout the body. How the movement of this energy helps regulate the chemicals in our brains and calms us. How the mantras have both psychological and physiological effects on our body. Ultimately, he said, chanting is not only for the benefit of oneself, but for the benefit of all beings. The energy carried by the sound vibrations within you flows outwards and towards infinity. Touching all.

Needless to say, I lost the rhythm a few too many times but overall, I surprised myself. The experience made me realise that any growth happens outside of our comfort zone. Building new connections in our brains, keeping us on our toes and developing a curiosity for anything new. There was also something about sticking to a discipline of repeating a string of words that freed my mind from focusing on my discomfort.

The time to wrap up was slowly approaching. Who would think that after a solemn meditation and chanting session, a Buddhist monk would crack a joke? It turned out to be one of the most valuable lessons I'd learned. One which will stick with me forever and reshape how I approach the way I want to live. I hope that it will spark the same desire in you.

Being with a monk was the perfect opportunity to ask about the elusive power of meditation. I've also always been curious about a monk's path towards enlightenment. Was I in the presence of an enlightened monk? After all, he must have been in his late sixties... My question was simple and straightforward: "Kuniatsu, what did meditation bring to your life?"

I am, of course, expecting the ultimate answer: enlightenment.

His reply caught me by surprise: "It keeps me out of trouble!" We both laughed.

Was he not on a personal journey to finding enlightenment? Had I been deceived? Was he really a monk? What kind of trouble did he mean?

Of course, I couldn't dare ask any of these silly questions. But then he said something seemingly insignificant yet surprisingly rich in meaning, "It gives me discipline so I can do what I enjoy."

He admitted that he was taken aback by my question. He'd never been asked before. I was equally taken aback by his answer.

It was time to make our way down the mountain. His words were like little seeds immediately taking roots in my mind. He asked if I preferred walking back on my own or with him. Despite wanting to spend more time with Kuniatsu, I knew that I had to go back alone. There were words I needed to ponder and meanings I needed to capture. I thanked him and told him that I was definitely meant to be there on that day. He agreed and added that not only was I meant to be there, but I was also meant to be with him on my own. We needed not say more.

Contemplating the forest as I slowly walked down, it felt even more mesmerising. This encounter was not random. This monk made me realise an expansive and liberating truth: Discipline leads to freedom.

Freedom to, freedom from.

Counterintuitive perhaps? Sounds insignificant? Does it mean freedom to do anything?

Discipline, a Host to Freedom

Freedom can mean different things to different people. Most often we associate it with freedom of speech, freedom of choice, our freedom under a democratic government.

Now, consider these more personal aspects:

Freeing yourself from the judgement of others which ultimately takes away your own power.

Finding freedom from a negatively serving addiction.

Freedom to devote energy towards what matters more to you.

Freedom from being shaken by external events.

It can also mean freeing yourself from getting drawn into your mind's whirlwind of thoughts and beliefs that can sometimes take over your life. With focus and practice, you can develop a greater sense of awareness and release damaging thoughts to make space for uplifting, constructive and compassionate thoughts.

With a deliberate discipline, you can free yourself from what is negatively impacting your health. A health conscious or fitness conscious discipline for your body can bring you freedom to move with joy and confidence. Freedom to participate in activities you felt you couldn't do. Freedom to feel good, to experience new possibilities. To go out more. Discipline, once you engage with it, will free space within to be filled with healing and renewed motivation. Whichever form it takes, you will feel free to live in harmony with yourself and the world around you. Engaging with a discipline is to connect with it. Ultimately, you will also feel more connected with yourself and free to experience more of you.

In the monk's case, his meditating discipline keeps him out of trouble, giving him the freedom to enjoy whatever it is he enjoys, and freedom from the actual thing(s) that he would otherwise fall prey to.

Every day as I prepare and eat breakfast, I listen to healing and positive affirmations that resonate with me. That's my waking up discipline. It may sound trivial, and that's pretty much how it felt at the beginning. But I had to find something, back then... The initial days and months following the news that my husband would go his own way were crushing. The grief held me prisoner and I needed to find any little help I could to free myself from the deep pain and the constant tornado of negative thoughts engulfing me.

This simple discipline of listening to meaningful affirmations is like a guide to readjusting our internal radio from negative self-talk to tuning into a positive and constructive self-talk frequency. A few weeks had passed and this practice became as necessary as my morning coffee. It gradually led me to experience freedom from being attached to recurring negative and self-defeating beliefs, replacing them with uplifting and kind thoughts towards myself. It also helped in my healing journey and cleared a mental path to welcoming peace in my heart and in other areas of my life.

It's been three years now and it feels like the people I enjoy listening to online have become part of my life. The by-products are immense.

There Are No Limits

This notion of discipline leading to freedom bears no frontiers. A few months ago, during Covid-19 lockdowns, I read a Facebook post from Troels Bager, professional dancer and three times world Latin-American champion, inviting dancers to an online class. He wrote:

"We'll look at how to use mechanics as a tool to, not only improve Your dancing, but to develop skills and create freedom within the restrictions."

I immediately noticed how he referred to the use of mechanics as a 'tool', hence, linking a discipline to something positive and constructive. He also associated other benefits to the manifestation of discipline: Developing skills and creating freedom.

His quote intrigued me and prompted me to reach out to him. I wanted to dig a little further into the topic of how he viewed discipline and freedom in his own life. Not only did he kindly accept to expand on those subjects but he also took this request to heart and shared some rich insights which we can all benefit from.

What do discipline and freedom mean for him?

Discipline and freedom become a way of life. While enjoying freedom as a well-earned reward, he actually realises how much the process is enjoyable. It develops as a path on which he continuously improves his skills and gains knowledge. This process becomes so fulfilling and satisfying that it inspires him to apply the same approach to other areas of his life. As such, freedom grows and expands in new ways.

DISCIPLINE → SKILLS BUILDING → FREEDOM

What are the challenges he faces along the way?

Comfort

Constantly making sure that comfort doesn't take over and dominate his choices and actions. Comfort can be sneaky, it can show up in disguise, or as doubts, insecurities, and use rational arguments to take back control. It may argue its case as to why you shouldn't stick to your plan and continue your journey of growth. We ought to be aware of this trap, focus on our goal and find ways to bypass comfort when it shows up.

Finding Satisfaction and Fulfilment Within the Discipline

Sticking to the discipline without feeling like its prisoner.

If it becomes a weight that drags us down, his advice is to commit to the process of skills building rather than focusing on an immediate sense of freedom. Relating what we do to how it will contribute to expanding our possibilities. Making the process count throughout. Discipline inherently implies a commitment, something long-lasting and fulfilling.

"Discipline has given me control and allowed me to build and enjoy freedom rather than search for freedom."

"Discipline has given me trust in who I am, what I can accomplish and how to face obstacles."

Troels Bager.

If you ever have the chance to watch him and his partner Ina dance, you'd not only see the absolute passion for their art but the effortless beauty and fluidity of their movements. Breathtaking freedom stemming from huge efforts and an incredible discipline.

The expansive space of discipline and freedom

When we engage in our chosen discipline, in our quest for the freedom we seek, we naturally set our expectations on the positive impact it will deliver in our life. But, an even greater realisation comes along the process: while working hard and overcoming our own doubts and temptations to give up the dream, we discover that our discipline delivers even greater results.

Our 'skills building', whether those skills are life skills or physical skills, not only lead us to our freedom goal but also compound over time, generating momentum to experiencing expanded freedom. We become increasingly motivated to apply these principles to other areas of our lives.

Inspiration

What is the freedom you hope for and why? Which discipline can you start adopting to achieve this freedom? What are the benefits you'd see manifest in your own life? You can too, experience the same benefits Troels did, whether it is a physical discipline or any other form of discipline.

Be clear in identifying what you want to achieve, why and how. You can seek advice if you need guidance on that path. Over time, your newly found freedom will cleanse and shape your thoughts, and your discipline will give you a sense of fulfilment and accomplishment. Your whole being will radiate harmony and confidence.

A smaller start with big results

If the thought of adopting a discipline is daunting, on the way to reaching your goal, start with something which doesn't require an initial massive amount of effort. Ideally, do it at the start of your day as a way set a positive tone to the rest of your day. You will get some satisfaction early on and motivation to carry on. Whatever you decide to do, put it in your daily schedule so as to give it the importance it deserves and so that it gets done, just like meetings.

Hold yourself accountable and take time to reflect on your progress. In a matter of a few days, you will already have gained enough momentum to experience how the freedom you desire is within reach. Celebrate the small steps just like the bigger accomplishments.

You will find what's ideal for your journey but if you need some inspiration, here are just a few simple ideas to explore:

Overall wellbeing

A daily meditation to free yourself from the noises or the insanely fast speed at which some events are unfolding. Spending time being with your breath, with yourself. With kindness.

Physical

Does your body need freedom to express itself with more ease and self-assurance? Do you feel restricted and trapped from having neglected your body, perhaps weight wise? Does it limit you, your encounters?

Could it be a physical discipline you ought to adopt?

If your physical body needs to find its optimal healthy zone, you could also, for example, learn how to cook for yourself (and your family). A discipline that would give you the freedom to choose what's best for your body and ultimately the freedom to explore what you have been reluctant to engage in.

Cultural

Since discipline implies skills building, why not learn the basics of the language spoken at your next destination? Essential language courses are readily available and easy to follow. You will have so much more freedom to explore the richness that lies outside tourists' areas, to address locals in their language and learn more of their ways.

Psychological

Social media captivity is something we all experience. We seem to experience more of its ugliness compared to the good it contributes to our lives. If you feel trapped in any shape or form, disengage from it to break free from its addictiveness, from the envy or passivity that it promotes. Disengage from the people and accounts that suck the most out of you or take periodic breaks for one hour a day, one day a week, one week a month. You will have the freedom to be in control of what you let in as opposed to being controlled by it. The freedom to be in charge as opposed to giving that power away to others and to social media platforms. The freedom to harness your own power.

Something else I'd like you to ponder: Do you hold on to recurring longings or thoughts you know to be inglorious? They also are agents of captivity. They keep you, your mind and your heart captive. What can you do for yourself or others while in captivity? Nothing. You can change that now.

What is the freedom you desire and why? Find a discipline which will lead you to it and stick to it. Freedom will come and endure.

Financial

Gaining financial knowledge for the freedom to confidently invest for your future. It can also offer you more freedom to give generously. Watch a YouTube video on the basics of investing a few times per week, or take a once-a-week online course.

No matter what you choose for yourself, there will be moments when your discipline will lapse and it's okay. You are not a machine. Press reset. That's already going to be a good discipline, reminding yourself that you are still in the game.

Discipline inherently and obviously requires us to do something over and again. The word 'again' is a powerful little mantra in itself which we can turn to daily. 'Again' is A-gain. Yes, **a gain**. Now and tomorrow.

Final Thoughts

Free yourself to be who you want to be.

The discipline you engage in will become part of you and build you. A key to the freedom you desire.

In spending time with nature,
one receives far more than he seeks.
Next time you are walking in the woods, appreciate what it does for your mind and body. Perhaps you will find in it something freeing, too.

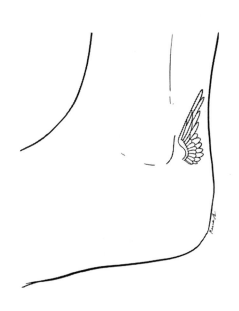

Chapter 2
Matterness and Gentleness

November 7, 2017.

"If ever I die, whoever finds this book, please have mercy on my broken soul. I ask for forgiveness. I ask for protection over my daughter, my husband, my family and friends. I shall be your guardian angel provided I make it to heaven." <3

Dire. And it's not the only note of that nature I have written in my life. The only reason why this one still exists is that it belongs in a beautifully gold-bound notebook my sister gave me as a Christmas present in 2014. It bears her love for me and it is one of the first things I pack in my carry-on whenever I travel.

All the other dark notes I wrote ended up shredded into unrecognisable pieces as if I thought that their vanishing would also mean that somehow the experiences of wanting to part with life would also vanish along; they don't. I have come to realise that they stay because those experiences have the power to make you grow and find healing.

At the peak of despair, my fervent prayers were addressed to the devil. I wanted him to come take me so I wouldn't have to do it myself. For not to die with the guilt of leaving my loved ones behind and causing immeasurable pain in their own lives. My pain would definitely end but what unthinkable pain would I leave for my daughter, husband and loved ones to carry for the rest of their lives?

My daughter, who knew about my previous struggles, once said to me in her soft voice: "Mommy, I need you, you will never leave me, promise?" Those words would forever be engraved in my heart. I felt selfish and besides, the sheer thought of taking my own life was so frightening. Yet, I desperately wanted to go. Sitting on that peak of despair though, someone was there to meet me, embrace me, weep with me, comfort me and save me. Just as those words from my daughter kept on replaying in my head.

As I laid in bed, in a flood of tears and trapped in emotions which now seem impossible to describe, my husband reached out for the Bible and randomly opened it to a Psalm. The one he landed on was all but random. It couldn't have been. The words were meant as a message to me. God knew.

With gentleness and love, he calmed me down. I felt safe in his arms. I felt God's presence through the words he read. Little did I know that this experience would have a deeper meaning. Life prepares us to surmount obstacles and navigate sharp changes of direction. It can guide us in our personal development journey and perhaps even in becoming someone's lifeline at critical times. Little did I know...

Years later I found myself on the receiving end of the most heart-breaking phone calls of my life. Even as I am writing these words, I can vividly recall the raw emotions that took over my body. The interstate was packed on my drive back home and I could most definitely not carry on a conversation despite being on hands-free so I quickly pulled over onto the shoulder. I knew it was real, so real, too real.

The words went something like this: "Mommy, I'm done with living, I can't anymore, it's over." With a pounding heart, the world felt like it was going to collapse, that the person I love the most was alone and defenceless on the edge of a precipice.

A dozen thoughts sprinted through my mind at lightning speed including getting out of my car and running all the way from Baltimore to Philadelphia to go and hold her. Getting back on the I-95 and doing a U-turn crossing eight lines of heavy traffic would not get me there on time either, most likely not at all. I didn't have three hours; she didn't have three hours. She only had the now and I only had her on the phone.

"Hey cocotte, I'm with you. Hang in there. I'm not going anywhere. I'm staying with you."

Calmness and gentleness, I thought.

I asked her short questions to keep her engaged, and let her know I was listening.

"Where are you now?"

Short questions, soft voice.

She spoke, and cried, and spoke.

"There's no hurry, I'm here, listening. You can cry, it's okay."

"Is there something that triggered that feeling?"

She spoke a little.

"It sounds overwhelming but we'll get you through this, I promise."

"I love you so much, we all love you so much and you are our sunshine."

"Your light is dim and down at the moment. I'll help you. By the time I get to Philly, it would be kind of late but I can look for a train for you to hop on and you can be home with me in D.C. soon and we will spend some time together."

"You've been through lots. Be gentle with yourself, you need a bit of time. You matter."

She was still listening and repeating words of distress.

"I'm not going anywhere…We will be together in a couple of hours."

Trying to buy some time.

"Can you ask a friend to accompany you to the train station?"

I wanted to make sure she'd get on the train.

I quickly logged onto Amtrak, talked through my search to keep her with me, found a train and that evening she was with me in Washington, D.C.

Her tender words from years ago became mine. In the taxi on the way home, as we held hands, I whispered: "Cocotte, I need you too, you will never leave me, promise?"

What saved her that day? God's love. His words and wisdom through me.

My daughter is my sunshine and despite the fact that she felt like her light was extinguishing, it still shone. The crushing events which had previously afflicted her undoubtedly found their way back to the surface of her being. Like sea creatures suddenly springing out from the ocean's depths.

We don't know what people are going through, which storms they may find themselves in. If you feel that you are sinking or riding stormy waters, remember that you are still the captain of your ship.

It takes an enormous amount of skill, courage and strength just to be at the wheel of your vessel and hold onto it so please, give yourself some credit. Be gentle and compassionate with yourself. You may need to ask help from your crew and rely on them until the storm passes.

Reach out to shipmates in your life. Shipmates are the captain's right hand. They support their captain, no questions asked. Shipmates can steer, stand watch, and navigate when the captain is not on duty. Read this again: the captain is not always on duty, nor are you. Your shipmates can also safely berth your ship.

When the waters calm, you will be able to enjoy riding the gentle waves together. If other storms approach, you will be better prepared, each time. You will learn how to recognise the signs, ask for help pro-actively and rely on that extra bit of confidence you are building up.

Remember that God's love will always be your anchor. You can pray to him and if you are not at a point where you can call on his name, it's okay, his love will manifest through the people you reach out to.

A few years later, after navigating another storm, my daughter sent us a picture of a delicate angel wing tattooed on her ankle. Her message read like this:

"I know you guys aren't fans of this kind of art, but I hope you agree this is a step up from the atrocity on my butt*. For me, a lovely tribute to someone who I wholeheartedly believe, through God, saved my life. And a reminder to keep running towards all the beautiful things ahead. Don't worry, last one for many, many, many years (didn't feel good...rewarded myself with a slice of Whole Foods pizza, which made me think of our Sunday afternoons after church in Bethesda and then went to the gym, hehehe)."

That someone was Madison Holleran, a freshman at the University of Pennsylvania. She died on Jan. 17, 2014, when she jumped off a rooftop of a parking garage near the campus. Madison was a wonderful, smart and beautiful young woman inside and out. She was cherished by her friends. Her Instagram account showed a successful and happy college student although, behind the scenes, the track athlete was struggling with her mental health. She was just 19.

My daughter was the same age, from the same university and was miraculously saved from ending her life in the same way by an angel sent by God. That angel was Madison Holleran.

Depression is not a one-size-fits-all condition. If happiness is a choice, depression is sometimes construed as a kind of weakness, a character flaw. Nothing could be further from the truth. It is so much deeper and more complex than that. Its existence lies in the web of brain chemistry, life circumstances and pressures, and that web can catch a prey with no mercy. My daughter said to me once: "I was not fighting for myself, but I was fighting for you and Daddy."

Whatever you are going through, the value of talking openly about one's innermost feelings and emotions can never be underestimated. If the words don't come to you at the time, take just a first step and reach out.

Whatever problems you are dealing with, know that there is a space within you that is free of all problems. In the deeper dimension of your being. Reach out for a hand to help you find it.

I believe that when you feel like nothing to yourself, alone, invisible or caught in a storm, God is your guiding light, high above the ocean's horizon. Even if you can't see

Him through the thick clouds, He is always there. He will shine upon you, comfort you and help you navigate a storm through the support of your shipmates, through the gentle words of a parent, a friend, a therapist or even the warm presence of your pet. When you feel like a burden or worthless, your value is always known to God and the ones who love and support you. They will guide you back onto course to realising your dream journey. When you don't have the words to cry, God listens to you and is praying for you. Let this remind you that you are seen, heard and deeply loved. You are known and you matter. You are not just matter and this is of great matter.

Let someone know today that they matter.
If you are the person who is struggling, reach out now,
you matter.

In turn, after you can safely anchor your ship, life may
use you to be someone else's lifeline.
What you have to offer also matters.

Here is a beautiful quote from a famous actor, above all a humble human being who's gone through storms of his own:

"If you have been brutally broken but still have the courage to be gentle to other living beings, then you're a badass with a heart of an angel."

Keanu Reeves.

Final Thoughts

A storm can shipwreck you at a place you didn't intend to.
Many pieces to pick up and reassemble. Much to discover.

The key is gentleness, because we all matter.

Remember:
'Storms get tired too'.
The Boy, The Mole, The Fox and The Horse,
Charlie Mackesy.

I dedicate this chapter to Caroline and Rachel and all of my daughter's friends who have been her shipmates and lovingly carried her to safety through her life's storms.

Part of the proceeds of this book will go to support the www.madisonholleranfoundation.org
*A tattoo which reads 'Made in Canada' accompanied by a maple leaf.

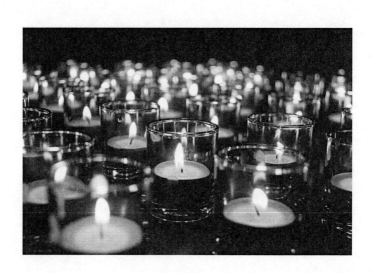

Chapter 3
One

The Intrinsic Value of One Lies in Its Infinite Magnitude

Have you ever felt inspired by heroes who do amazing things to make the world a better place only to be demoralised by the thought of not having what they have to do the same? Do you find yourself thinking you are not doing anything worthwhile enough because you are not volunteering in a refugee camp or raising huge sums of money for a charity? These questions certainly prompt us to reflect about our impact in the world. The necessary question though is: What is your role number **ONE**?

One thing I love to do when travelling is to spend quiet time sitting in the pews of a church. Praying, appreciating the grandeur and architecture, and wondering what kinds of prayers are filling the sacred space. Catholic churches and basilicas especially attract me; their walls holding a distinctive scent, which, for me, is synonymous with God's presence. I came to appreciate the lingering musty and musky smell from incense, filling the air with an aromatic illusion of burning smoke. It's as if there is an ethereal quality to it.

Whilst at church, the tradition of lighting votive candles is one I cherish. I see it as a humble gesture that seals a prayer, symbolising the union between our heart and God's. Sitting in the pews of Old St Patrick's Basilica today in SoHo, I had a little moment of epiphany thinking of this incessant questioning about my reach and role in the world.

We all desire to make a difference while we're alive. How can I contribute to empower others? Heroes' stories were scrolling in my head. Thinking about the incredible (and some really creative!) achievements from ordinary people during the pandemic, lifting people up from making ends meet or making sure the vulnerable were being cared for. The list goes on. One common thread united them: They acted by taking one step. They went for ONE. They took action, just one to start. They took part in the play. They went for the role. Their role.

It dawned on me as I struck a long matchstick to light a candle for each person I was praying for, that one match was enough to light many candles. A much too simple and obvious fact you might think, and it is. Yet, its meaning is profound. One minuscule flame was enough to spread light, to ignite many more. And so it is with how every day heroes make a difference.

Have you ever struck a match, watching the flame slowly burn down, and just as it neared your skin, quickly blew it out? I can most definitely relate to that. When our match reaches that point, blackened and useless, how can it bring light? Is the moment when the flame starts to burn our skin an obvious sign that we ought to do something with our light rather than blow it out? We can all be observers, let our match burn down and blow the flame out. Slowly, it gets at us. We feel the discomfort. Why? As human beings, we are meant to serve. We are made from the same source, we breathe the same air, we are all interconnected.

> *"Selflessness is the surest route to inner peace and a meaningful life. Selflessness heals the self."*
> Jay Shetty, Think Like A Monk

Connect and Create

> *"We are nature and if we look at and observe nature carefully, nature is always serving. The sun provides heat and light. Trees give oxygen and water. Water quenches our thirst. They (trees) live solely for the benefit of others. They tolerate wind, rain, heat and snow, but still provide shelter for our benefit. The only way to be one with nature is to serve. It follows that the only way to align properly with the universe is to serve because that's what the universe does."*
> Jay Shetty, Think Like A Monk

To this I would like to add that nature is also always creating and hence provides us with another model for realising this connectedness. By serving, we create. We create hope, connections, better living environments, and new opportunities.

What we become, we create. By becoming agents of change, we create change. By becoming agents of peace, we create peace. By becoming agents of love, we create more love.

Achievements in the external world are only possible through achievements in our internal world. Service changes our internal world and benefits all of whom we are connected to. From finding ourselves being consumed with worries and all kinds of 'stuff', to serving instead, we create harmony within us and around us. From finding ourselves consuming our time and energy on social media 'stuff', to serving instead, we find ourselves creating meaningfulness within and around us.

We have access to a life-long supply of matches we can use to pursue our compassionate goals. We are given these many chances by the grace of God.

We live in a world where many hold an unlit candle. Perhaps they are mourning the death of a loved one. Maybe they lost their job, are heartbroken or in a struggling marriage. Perhaps they are depressed, sick or lonely. Look around you, ask.

There will always be 'big' heroes, making a huge impact. There will also be 'little' heroes, making a big difference in one person's life. Both started with one person to care for, one idea they brought to life, one phone call, one post, etc. Some had big dreams or some may not even have a dream, yet they all started with impacting the life of one person and inspired others to do the same. They connected with one or many and they created for one or many.

From One to an Expanded Reach

Years ago, through an opportunity to deliver meals to people in need, I met a person who would have a big impact in my life without him ever realising to which extent. He was an older gentleman living on his own, in near absolute poverty. There was something utterly eccentric about him that initially intimidated me. Very thin and tall, he had an unhealthy ghost-like complexion, not so attractive teeth and was always dressed in the most eclectic and dandy-like deeply used clothes. Huge rings adorned his fingers and a bunch of chunky long chains with odd pendants hung from his skinny neck. His name was Mr P. He lived in a tiny corner room at the back of a run-down house set back from the road, quite deep in the woods. It felt like a place where a horror movie could have been filmed: eerie and dark with tall trees keeping the sunlight away. There was a 'no trespassing' metal sign midway down the driveway to deter people from approaching the house. I learned much later that the old gentleman who owned the house had put it there so that volunteers like me wouldn't come too close to his house. I still wonder why...

It definitely felt most uninviting and I had to stick by this bizarre rule that I was not to knock on Mr P.'s door but rather, sit in the car, call him and wait until I saw him walk down the driveway to meet him halfway. Knowing that most people we served were also lonely or sick, what was I to do to get to know Mr P. and offer him a little more than a meal?

Have you read the book, *The Little Prince*? Despite not having understood its meanings when I read it as a child, the story came back to life while thinking of how to befriend Mr P. At the time, I'd found the book a bit creepy and I was now finding myself feeling rather uncomfortable and unwelcome.

After a couple of weeks of progressively longer chats, it became obvious that Mr P. was clearly well educated and travelled. He recited poetry and told me tales of his youth while living in Africa as a son of a diplomat. He had later dressed windows at Bloomindales in NYC and acted in Shakespeare's plays. Little by little, our story felt more and more like that of the Little Prince and the fox's. The fox who had taught the Little Prince that the important things in life are visible only to the heart, and that love makes a person responsible for the beings that one loves.

As the months went by, we would both be looking forward to our long conversations, I'd bring him flowers with a rolled-up poem or a prayer he could read in bed at night. I no longer had to call him from my car, he knew I was coming and would wait for me halfway down the driveway. He had quit smoking, was eating all of his food, took walks to and from the road for half an hour every day. He proudly combed his hair and shaved his sparse grey beard before my arrival. We'd find a sunny spot to stand in through the thickness of the woods on cold winter days. It didn't matter if it was raining or freezing.

It is said that by being tamed, in the case of the fox, something went from being ordinary to special and unique. That is the beauty coming from doing something good for ONE person.

"He was a soldier of joy. If his sufferings were manifold so were his delights," his sister said. Mr P.'s acting days were long gone. He was now playing his life's role: Joyfully connecting to everyone he met and always seeing them off on a cheerful note. The physical and mental illness he bore for so long ravaged his body, yet he never complained. He had immense empathy and often quoted from Plato: "Be kind, for everyone you meet is fighting a hard battle."

He would pray for me when I needed healing. He had opened the door to his minuscule one-bedroom apartment to proudly show me the hundreds of trinkets he had collected during his many trips around the world. Some were

46

collectables to rival museum pieces. Pages of poetry he wrote overflowed from disgruntled shoe boxes.

Months passed or was it two years? I can't remember. One Friday morning in the spring of 2015, as I pulled in the long driveway, Mr P. was not there. I decided to call him and he did not pick up. Reluctantly, I left his bagged meal, groceries and a little bouquet on his doorstep and called the charity to let them know he didn't seem to be home. A few days later, I received an email from his beloved sister. Mr P. had passed away.

In his eulogy, she wrote: "Oscar Wilde says a cynic is a person who knows the cost of everything and the value of nothing. Mr P. was the reverse of this: He knew the cost of nothing and the value of everything."

His suffering was immense. He drowned in the glory of nature and literature. His relationships with people were singular because he looked at the world with his new eyes every day. He was flamboyant in generosity and love.

Who befriended whom in the end? Mr P. did more for me than I ever did for him. His impact on the one me would not die when he left.

My true wish with this book is that it will help at least one person. In at least one way. Change one person's day, or life, for the better. And, that the flow of life will carry it as far as it belongs.

Our Role, Our Time to Act

As we said earlier, when we think about how we can make a difference, we often fall for the myth that what we need to be doing something on a large-scale or that we ought to have enough time or money to serve. If you are like me, and so many others, you might think that the difference you can make is insignificant and even quit at the thought of it. Just as light spreads though, one action will lead to another, and you may not even be able predict the outcome. In becoming intentional about our impact, our role becomes increasingly clear.

What was fascinating and most inspiring during the pandemic was witnessing how many ordinary people set out with one idea, one video or one lap across a garden to finding themselves inspiring their neighbours, and even the whole country. ONE's magnitude is infinite.

The step that is easily overlooked when trying to make a difference is the acting part. We aim, overthink and procrastinate. We wait to have just that extra bit of time or money. Or we strike a match and let it die down. We must focus our energy into achieving something small first rather than deliberating about the outcome. It is said that creative people are not hung up on fixed definitions of what any form of reality may be. They are not limited by molds.

You are inherently creative, we all are. We are part of nature, creating and serving. Ignite one person's candle first. If your matchstick is longer, you can extend your reach. The light and the flow of good energy will find a path to carry your action until infinity and will also nourish your own life. Service connects us, nurtures gratitude and compassion, and give us a sense of meaning and purpose.

"The more grateful we feel, the happier we become. This is because gratitude helps us realise we are all connected. Nobody feels like an island when feeling grateful. Gratitude awakens us to the truth of our interdependent nature."

Haemin Sunim

The Things You Can See Only When You Slow Down.

All of us already do good around us. Some already have plans to shoot for the stars and transform our world. There are infinite examples to keep us going personally, and for the betterment of humanity. Regardless of the scope, the common denominator is acting. Making it a way of life.

"But remember that whatever you are giving was given to you. When you pass it on, you can't take credit for it."

Jay Shetty, Think Like a Monk

Who Will Sit in the Pews?

A few years ago, I read a passage in a self-help book which I noted as follows: Life is merely unpredictable that we should be able to write our obituary today in order to see if we are truly living or merely existing. We should ask ourselves how many people will attend our funerals to measure our worth and make sure we live every moment.

I don't know about you but in stumbling upon that note and giving it more thought, I must say that I have a real issue with these statements.

How does one even measure his/her/their worth? Do you live your days with the content of your obituary in mind? Do you need to know how many people will sit in the pews? Does more means that you have lived a better life?

Yes, we need to truly live, and not merely exist. What we do connects us to others, makes us more grateful and also gives us a sense of purpose. When we pursue compassionate goals, we necessarily shift our focus towards appreciation. It builds positive energy within and around us. We need to think about our role, our impact, and act. We need to use our matches whilst they are lit.

If one person sits in the pews, that person is a light you lit. A life saved, a heart healed or a gift of friendship. An inspiration to do the same for someone else.

If the pews are filled, all will rejoice at having been in the presence of your light. Your light will have lifted many out of darkness, energised others, and perhaps even transformed the world. Making it a brighter place.

"Do not wait for leaders; do it alone, person to person."
Mother Teresa

"If your actions inspire others to dream more, learn more, do more and become more, you are a leader."
Simon Sinek, Leaders Eat Last:
Why Some Teams Pull Together and Others Don't.

Final Thoughts

Can you think of a memorable act of kindness that was extended to you? How did it change you or your life?

How will you use your light every day?
*What is your role number **one**?*

***Act** in that role every day.*
That's going to be the key to your legacy.

This chapter is dedicated to my dear friends Sara and the late Mr P. Both selflessly and lovingly extended their light to shine into my life. I am sharing it with all of you.

Parts of the proceeds will be donated to foodandfriends.org.

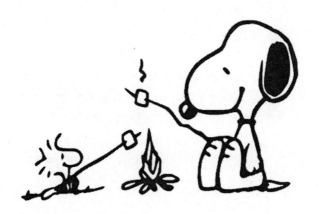

Chapter 4
Full Presence
Superman and the Marshmallow

Have you ever sat by your computer or phone waiting for one beep that would make it all better, a miracle beep, a reply to your 'I am sorry' message? To something you've said or done, or perhaps not said nor done? Or any other much anticipated reply? Sitting in front of my computer, writing to you, that is precisely what I am waiting for. I had hurried, hurdled over my better conscience, and now, I am paying the price. Can you relate?

The plan was to use my quarantine time in Montreal to make progress on this book, catch up with family and friends daily, and stay fit physically and mentally. The pandemic drove most of us onto unchartered territories, pulling us in many directions, allowing us to revisit, refine and even redefine our lives.

From the small fireplace in my hotel room, timeless flames seem to be speaking to me. There is such a fine line between their ever-comforting warmth and their ruthless intensity. They will burn you in a split second if you don't pay attention, if you don't approach them with care and respect a safe distance. Many of you will have had the joy of roasting, over a campfire, a soft marshmallow at the end of a long stick and of savouring its sweet, melted centre after having eaten the golden crisp bubbly outer layer. It required finesse and patience to roast the perfect marshmallow and presence to enjoy the delightful process. They were lots of times when we were so eager to eat it that we just couldn't wait and held the tip of our stick so close to the flames that the marshmallow would catch fire. The outside became charred black and the centre wouldn't have had time to melt yet. It was a big disappointment each time!

A Presence in Flames

Many years ago, whilst my daughter was in her early teens, I remember being drawn to a little notebook she had left on her desk. Curiosity's strong grip got a hold of me and I couldn't resist but take a peek. Needless to say, it was a terrible mistake and I got burned. Not just a surface burn, a second-degree burn. I had, above all, wounded my daughter's trust in me. It must have felt like a moral violation that cut deep through the core of her young soul.

We both sat on her bed after the initial shockwave had somewhat dissipated. I profusely apologised and told her that I wish I were Superman. Superman, flying faster than the speed of light, making the Earth turn back in time, reversing the course of events. Turning back time and leaving her notebook to rest on her desk, safely holding her young wonders and experiences. Turning back time to where her trust in me was whole. Turning back time to actually take time to consult with my conscience before reaching for her journal.

Those were the words she uttered: "Mommy, if you were Superman and could go back in time, you'd never learn from your mistakes." Of course, we have all heard those words but when they spontaneously come from a twelve-year-old, you take notice. A child's wisdom is so pure. Not only had she forgiven me, but she had also given me her gift of unconditional love. That gift of love which endures beyond forgiveness, healing relationships. Letting me off the hook, loving me, including my flaws. These noble traits define her beauty to this day.

Presence Is a Catalyst for Trust

Presence and trust share a strong connection. Being fully present anchors us, and compels us to add meaningfulness to what we do for the other whether they are around or not. We make choices with integrity; we strive to serve the other and nurture this connection. If it loosens, being present prompts us to question ourselves. Our presence is a catalyst for building, maintaining and even growing trust. Trust holds relationships together. It deepens our relationships. It allows us to feel safe so that we can be vulnerable enough to emotionally connect with another person. It is an unspoken code of honour. As trust grows, if we break it, we sever its ties not only with the other person but very often with ourselves. Presence is a catalyst for building trust, and trust is a building block to love.

Often times, we rush through the living nature of our relationships.

"Regret for the things we did can be tempered with time; it is regret for the things we did not do that is inconsolable."

1951 January 5, Akron Beacon Journal, Syd Cannot Stand Christmas Neckties by Sydney J. Harris, Quote Page six, Column five, Akron, Ohio. (Newspapers.com).

Presence as a Relationship Choice

Presence not only encourages engaging conversations but in choosing to be aware of how we communicate with one another and how we listen to one another, we discover. We discover ways forward together. We discover more about the evolving nature of our relationship. We observe its intricacies. They provide a gateway to connecting us together far beyond the surface.

We choose to notice and remember. We remember what matters most to them, what they are concerned about, we remember to ask. We anchor ourselves in the moment to see the other's point of view, to stand in their shoes. We pick up on warning signs, such as hard feelings, and we choose to address them rather than let them build. We mutually diagnose and heal. Presence is having our heads out of the sand, where we can clearly see. In paying attention, it also connects us to our conscience and illuminates our actions.

Sadly, I will live with the memory of having been so consumed by built-up resentment that, at the time when my husband returned from a climbing trip in the Himalayas, I didn't even ask him to see his pictures. To sit down and listen to his stories even if I had already seen loads of them on social media. This lack of presence sliced too deep. I not only failed him but failed myself. Could having cultivated this notion of full presence over the years lead to a different future? Of course, the 'coulds' and 'shoulds' and 'what ifs' are futile although the lessons remain.

Can you think of instances where your full presence clearly lacked, and what it resulted in? Can you also think of a time where it contributed to particularly joyful memories?

When we consciously pay attention, we choose a 'purpose moment'. In this moment, we are present with purpose and create connection with purpose.

Presence Creates Peace Within Ourselves

We often hurry to write a message which we regret right after pressing 'send'. We may have written it to feel better about ourselves or about a situation, and in the end, the opposite happens. The same happens with the things we say, wishing we could take back our words right after they left our tongue. An old-time friend of mine characterised this in a direct and humoristic way: "I say what I think and mean. I read the room first but there are words and time for certain discussions. I also let time pass to reflect rather than let my giant Amygdala ruin more...for me."

Reflect rather than regret.

When we deliberately reflect, we create a 'purpose moment' for ourselves; to ponder our words, written or spoken, so that they carry wisdom, humility and compassion. At peace with them and with ourselves.

Presence Creates Memories

In a 'purpose moment', we can choose to keep our phone in our bag and still capture the essence of what we are seeing in all of its angles and depths. Remembering to remember the scenery, sounds, images and words. We can revisit the experience in our minds and heart. Without a date and time stamp, this richness will be still accessible, in another form. Try a *purpose moment* today to replace a *phone moment* and choose to remember. When we choose to remember, we remember.

Presence Is a Gateway to Discoveries and Opportunities

In a 'purpose moment', we learn, for example, what a piece of art is telling us and not just what is it showing us. Seeing the 'big picture' gives us a good sense of the theme, of whether or not it is pleasing to us, etc. But it's often in observing something from a different angle, from a different distance, where discoveries happen. We uncover the nuances, the layers of colours, the objects and symbols we hadn't noticed at first glance. We see a story behind the shapes and figures. We come to appreciate what the piece is evoking in us.

Presence is a choice and a teacher.
You are who you choose to be.

Since I began to write, the flames have died down and I'm finding myself still waiting for that miracle beep from my phone. Earlier that day, I experienced yet another time where my presence was caught in that fire, engulfed in the flames of my own life circumstances, of my own agenda. I would be no Superman today either but, yet again, I embraced the lesson. A gain. That's how we grow. Constantly learning to be more present.

Who and What Can Teach Us to be More Present?

A master of a teacher on four legs

A few days after arriving in NYC to visit my daughter and meet her dog, she went on a trip that had recently been planned. The deal was that I'd look after her puppy in my hotel room for seven days. I was super excited about it but also very nervous.

Looking like a complete buffoon, portable crate in one hand, his home-away bag filled with toys and food on my shoulder, a brown paper shopping bag with his weewee pad and bowls on the other, and the little pup attached to a leash triple knotted around my forearm (I was afraid of losing him!), I hustled along the road all the way to my hotel. Arriving in my room, half dead, the brown paper bag half ripped and barely holding the stuff, I let him off the leash and he started doing something I had never witnessed before! In a panic, I Googled the 'symptoms' and it was something called the 'zoomies'. That little ball of energy was sprinting up and down the room at lightning speed, around the bed, under the bed and in between the table legs for about five minutes non-stop. He eventually calmed down, a little. I clearly needed to take the time to learn his ways and make him feel comfortable in this new place that wasn't home, without his mommy (aka my daughter). We survived a week together and by the end, just like when my daughter was little, he would fall asleep in my arms. I would stay there, not moving an inch (despite pins and needles in my legs and desperately having to go to the bathroom), observing him, noticing his little twitches, laughing at his snoring, and caressing his velvety head. It was heaven.

We ended up spending four months together. He'd become my afternoon buddy while my daughter was at work. He made me appreciate and see things I had not paid attention to before. I learned to recognise his likes and dislikes, and cute habits. To recognise when he needed his freedom. I also learned more about myself.

On one of our last days together before my flight back to London, we headed to his favourite spot on the corner of Pearl and Dover streets. The fog had descended over Brooklyn Bridge giving it an enigmatic allure. There was something eerie in the air that day. Something was different, even the look in his eyes. He ran with his usual frantic energy from one end of the dog run to the other, zooming underneath the cold metal benches, but, alas, none of his friends were there. I could see the disappointment and sadness in his big, beautiful eyes. He sat, without prompting, looking at me.

The leash back on, we made our way towards Seaport and walked along the East River shore. As I trailed behind (he is by definition a pug but could pull a sleigh just like a Huskie!), I could but only marvel at this little bundle of joy trotting at full pace with his floppy shiny ears, loving to chase pigeons.

Back at my daughter's apartment after nearly two hours of walking, I was hoping I could get him to fall asleep as I was a bit exhausted and didn't really feel like playing fetch. It usually takes some clever manoeuvring around the apartment just to catch him. My strategy was to sit on the floor against the sofa by the round coffee table and block him as he tried to go around! I mean, if I didn't, he'd honestly play for hours on.

That afternoon though, everything was different. He knew, I am convinced of that. There have been too many signs since the beginning of the pandemic that this little black pug was more than a little black pug. After years of longing and waiting, my daughter received a call exactly one month before the lockdown closed in on all of us to say that a black puppy pug needed a home. The timing of his arrival was no coincidence; he was going to save her life when sickness and lockdown pressures hit hard.

I did not have to corner him as I sat on the cold wooden floor, my back leaning against the couch. He walked around the table, quietly sat beside me and rested his little head against my right arm. He did not move. I did not move. Tears rolled down my cheeks. It's as if he was saying: "I love you and I'll miss you." I stayed there with him, fully committed to this precious moment, appreciating the blessing.

He had been present with me all along and he had taught me the value of being present with him all along. I wish that one day he will sit next to me by a campfire, roasting the perfect marshmallow.

Grand little teachers

Children can teach us so much about presence without their conscious realisation. Some of my most treasured moments were when my newborn daughter would fall asleep in my arms after drinking her bottle of milk. Even though plenty of chores awaited me, every single time, I'd sit there, at times for hours, looking at her until she'd wake up. No phone. Not only looking at her but feeling her warmth, observing how she was changing from day to day, caressing her soft hair and hands, getting to know what made her feel comfortable or not. Only in those moments of being truly present can we really connect with and appreciate the reality in front of us. Only then can we notice and delight in all of its layers.

Children teach us 'purpose moments'. Through the purity of their interactions, their wonder for the people and the world. Make a point of observing children and ask yourself what you can learn from them.

Life's art studio

Next time you find yourself in a museum, gallery, or garden spend a few 'purpose moments' with the art you are standing before. Up close and away. Seeing things from a different perspective will also change the perspective within you. It expands our views.

There is no inherent meaning in a picture, drawing, or flower. We give it meaning. We create the meanings. Just as with pretty much everything in life!

Time

Everything happens at such fast pace that this speed becomes engrained in our active nature. Have you suffered the repercussions of acting hastily? I surely have, many times. The best tool we have is to embrace time. It's always there and we only have to remind ourselves of that simple word.

Curbing our enthusiasm to hurry by welcoming a bit more time can dramatically lead to better outcomes and certainly a greater sense of peace within ourselves (of course I am not talking about urgent things that require an immediate action from us). Would dedicating a little extra time add value to what you are about to do? Add value to someone's life?

And of course,

Meditation definitely comes to mind as it teaches us the value of pausing, breathing and becoming familiar with ourselves and our surroundings. We can also find moments during our day, without any interruptions, to just pay attention. and breathe.

One of my favourite meditation experts whom I've come across with online, Emily Fletcher, said two things I found very meaningful:

"The more you meditate, the less likely you are to make a mistake."

"You don't meditate to become good at meditating, but you mediate to become good at life."

Reflect on how much truth these statements hold. Can you also think of times where you have rushed through or rush to, and got burned?

Or times when you felt so calm and present that you knew it saved you from making a mistake? Of course, we learn through mistakes but our aim is obviously to get better at life.

By always remembering to take a step back, we can then move forward with full focus, attention and intention. There will be more to appreciate, more to contribute to and more reasons for our relationships to thrive. Befriending the stillness within us, at the centre of our being, is a key to keeping us present. It's worth keeping.

There is an old Zen proverb that says: "The only zen you'll find at the top of the mountain is the zen you bring with you."

What are your preferred sources for keeping you present? For accessing the zen within you? Are there more you would like to explore?

Final Thoughts

Being present is also knowing when to step back.

Indulge in that delicious marshmallow you roasted. With your full attention. That's the key.

Make your presence glow. Create your future through the present moment.

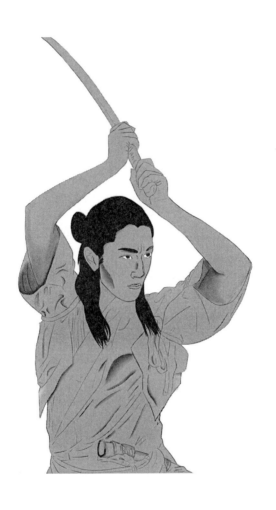

Chapter 5
Preparedness and Intuition
Where Inner Calm Meets the Target

Taking me through residential back alleys of Tokyo, the Uber driver dropped me off at the address provided. The destination didn't look anything like the picture from the website and despite his best efforts to help, the language barrier meant that I was left to finding my way on foot on my own. The neighbourhood's streets felt devoid of life. Not a soul in sight. Eventually, I stumbled upon an open courtyard breaking from rows of narrow indistinguishable residences attached to one another. Reluctantly, not wanting to trespass, I made my way through the open gates, attracted by the austere look of a neglected shrine in the distance. I pulled up the picture saved on my phone and indeed I was at the right place. Hesitantly, I circled the courtyard looking for a sign of life. A tall, poised man, the looks of a movie star, greeted me from the unassuming building's entrance adjacent to the shrine. It was really him, the samurai, and that was *the* temple.

In a surprisingly good English, he showed me the way upstairs where our workshop was to take place. Meticulously arranged on the bamboo floor mats were traditional training uniforms 'keikogi' of various colours and sizes. His assistant invited me to choose one and guided me to the small changing room. Excitement and nervousness were building up inside me as other people started to arrive. All in pairs, except for two men who had, just like me, decided to explore a more intimate side of the Japanese culture on their own.

The samurai invited us to kneel on the tatami around the massive 'chabudai'. I was wondering who would have sat around this gorgeous dark wooden table back in the times. There must have been so many stories embedded in its pores. Despite the somewhat half functioning noisy AC unit you could hear a pin drop. All eyes were on the samurai, explaining how our afternoon would unfold. As per the customary Japanese way of welcoming of guests, we were offered fragrant matcha tea and delicate sweets.

There was something about him. The elegancy and softness in the way he moved and spoke. His soft yet piercing glance. It's as if he was totally with us but also immersed in his own skin and being. He commanded our full attention. The story about his life as a pure descendent of a samurai was fascinating. With pride he drew his katana, the famous curved sword and one which had probably travelled many battlefields throughout the generations. It is said that the samurai's sword is his soul. Each part came alive as he ran his long slim fingers along its sharp edge, clearly indicating that it ought to be treated with great reverence. Above being a weapon, the katana is a symbol of a samurai's caste: A reminder of who he is, of his obligations and rights. I think it was an act of immense generosity on his part when he passed his sword around the table for each of the eight guests to observe and feel. Of course, there had to be one person who had to handle it against the firm instruction not to touch the sharp blade! It was the same guy who would obviously put on a show during the hands-on part of the workshop. An international jiu-jitsu champion with a stature synonymous to one of an imposing bodyguard for the rich and famous.

Before we would all get a go at handling our own sword and facing our opponent, the samurai proceeded to demonstrate his sword skills. After collecting his thoughts behind closed eyes, along with long deep breaths, he masterfully drew his sword from his scabbard and performed a sequence of steps and graceful moves. I felt transported back to the Edo period, just imagining how he could have been the last samurai! One could admire how years of practicing his art culminated in such a mesmerising and powerful demonstration. The blade slashed through thin air and with each slice, we could hear what would have been the sound of approaching doom. 'Tachikaze' or 'sword wind' is like a sharp whistling sound, a guaranteed sign of an ensuing perfect straight cut. He went on to decisively and sharply halve the 'Tameshigiri' (rolled tatamis) in lieu of an opponent, of course! The top half flung across the room with such velocity that I couldn't but imagine what happened a few centuries ago on the battlefield.

The art of the sword encapsulates both a physical and a spiritual dimension. The education of a samurai was influenced by Zen Buddhism in which the aim of Zen, applied to the mastery of the sword, was to make a samurai's thought and action instantaneous and live in togetherness. In *The Zen Way to the Martial Arts,* Zen master, *Taisen Deshimaru* told the story of a samurai who had just made a pilgrimage to the shrine of Hachiman, the Japanese god of war, in Kamakura at the midnight hour. Leaving the sacred precincts, he sensed a monster hiding behind a tree, waiting to pounce on him. Intuitively he drew his sword and slew it in the instant; the blood poured out and ran along the ground. He had killed it unconsciously. Intuition and action springing forth at the same time.

Striking without thinking was at the heart of instruction with the sword. For a samurai to hesitate ever so slightly before striking would mean giving his opponent time to deal the mortal blow. The samurai is not holding anything in his mind except the task at hand. He diligently and relentlessly practices until the wielding of the sword becomes second nature to him.

In his book, Samurai Strategy, Thomas Hoover writes: "He (Yukio Mishima) claimed that the perfect stroke must be guided toward a void in space, which, at that instant, your opponent's body will enter. In other words, your enemy takes on the shape of that hollow space you have envisioned, assuming a form precisely identical with it."

Learning about the samurai principles, which lie at the core of their heightened sixth sense, has helped me to see how intuition can most definitely be a skill to hone as opposed to something to shy away from. One of the most significant words from the excerpt above is 'guided'. His perfect stroke is guided towards a void in space.

What does it mean for us when we talk about using our intuition?

Using our intuition is not going about life with the feeling of being blindfolded or acting aimlessly. We can rely, consciously or unconsciously, on years of experience and knowledge. I think of it as 'preparedness'. Just like the samurai has been refining his skills and understands what he stands and fights for, our internal guidance is solidly built on our experiences, core values and principles. All of those amount to patterns that we come to recognise; consciously or unconsciously.

Have you ever made a decision and immediately started to feel sick, sweaty or uneasy? Could it have been your body's way of telling you that the decision your analytical mind came to is at odds with your instincts? Or, at odd with the values you stand for?

What can you do?

Stand on Your Benchmark

By mentally 'checking' if your decision or action is 'guided' or flows in accordance with your benchmark of core values and principles, you will come to use and trust your intuition with increasing curiosity.

> *"Intuition is a very powerful thing, more powerful than intellect."*
> *Steve Jobs*

By becoming one with your core values and principles, you are creating the firm ground upon which you can stand when you need to rely on your intuition. You are developing something within you as opposed to relying on the outer world to feed you.

What are your benchmark values and principles? It is a worthwhile exercise to do.

Say you are considering a seemingly alluring job offer and yet, something inside you tells you that it might not be the right thing to do. By having your core values and principles firmly established, whether it turns out to have been the right choice or not will actually not matter so much. You will have the peaceful reassurance that you acted in accordance with what lies at the centre of your being.

We have all asked ourselves, "Should I, or shouldn't I?" when having to accept or decline an invitation or when faced with a dilemma, for example. Many times, you may have said yes to something that felt wrong and made you feel physically uneasy. Did you go against your principles?

In the event that you stumble or the result is apparently opposite to what you anticipated, use it as an opportunity to sharpen your instincts by noticing what mistakes you made and how they made you feel. Refine your experiences, solidify your benchmark.

Be Prepared

The samurai's approach also teaches us the immense value of being prepared. With years of practicing sword skills, he focuses on the action rather that the technicalities. Being prepared involves practicing your skills, little by little every day. Finding ways to incorporate them as much as possible in what you do, whether they are physical or intellectual. Practicing them with intention and calmness. When the time comes to use your intuition, it will be your turn to strike with confidence.

Spot the Red Flags

Red flags are precisely that: Red flags! Often, we see them, sense them, and our intuition tells us 'don't go there' or it raises concerns within us. At times, we choose to ignore them and make up our own excuses, or lower our standards, to justify our decisions. Practice observing, feeling and questioning how your body reacts in various situations and what your mind tells you. Do not fool yourself.

See red flags as blessings, next time they come up! Seriously, do! Even if it's tempting to over rationalize, you will thank yourself later for sticking to your principles, for trusting your intuition.

Practice Being Aware of Patterns

Over the years, through your vast array of experiences and the knowledge you have gained from them, you come to recognise patterns and their meanings. For example, from different tones of voices, from the energy a crowd emits, from the ways people looks at you, from observing a group of people's behaviours, etc. Add those patterns to your internal compass.

We all have it.

Different writers give the word 'intuition' a great variety of meanings, ranging from direct access to unconscious knowledge, unconscious cognition, inner sensing, inner insight to unconscious pattern-recognition, and the ability to understand something instinctively, without the need for conscious reasoning.[4][5] source: Wikipedia

No matter how we describe it, we all have it. We have all had intuitive experiences. We are all intuitive. Invest in establishing solid core principles for your life. Nurture your deep confidence in them.

When you tap into your intuition, it also adds another dimension to unleash your creativity. Developing your intuition is like learning any new skill. The more you practice, the better you get at it. Be curious with it. Use your intuitive key!

Speaking of practice, it was now our turn to get a go at swinging our katana. From vertical overhead to horizontal and diagonal striking techniques, we all had great fun learning those new skills with our smoothed-edge swords. I was paired up with a bubbly guy from California who kept coming back to Japan out of pure love for the country and its people. With the whole of my petite frame lost in the oversized uniform, I pulled out the long sword and swung the blade. There was a moment of silence and then came the distinctive '*tachikaze*' whistling sound as it sliced through the air. Beginner's luck? Most likely since next came the slicing of the upright tatami roll or 'pretend enemy' and I massively botched it! Had it been the real enemy, I would have been the very unlucky one.

Taking a journey back in time that evening, reflecting on the samurai's inner calm and strength, I realised that the times I went against my intuition were when I was utterly distracted or did not have an unshakable confidence in my core values, principles and accumulated experiences. Nor did I listen to how my body felt. At other times, I tried to justify what I knew did not sit quite right. Have you ever experienced such feelings and/or situations?

Being undisturbed and prepared made the samurai confident in his life-long sharpened intuitive skills. Let that inspire us to practice and refine our own skills.

Final Thoughts

"The intuitive mind is a sacred gift and the rational mind is a faithful servant. We have created a society that honours the servant and has forgotten the gift." – Albert Einstein

Our intuitive key can open many doors and close others.

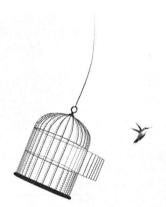

Chapter 6
Forgiveness
A Story with Wings

Unless one is a fervent bird lover, one wouldn't go all the way to Kenya to watch birds, right?

My hate-love relationship with birds started when I was very young, at a time when my parents took my sister and me on a road trip along Canada's east coast with Iles-de-la-Madeleine as the end destination. One day, we spent countless hours in the car heading out to visit a bird sanctuary in Gaspésie, nesting site to a colony of some 100,000 huge white migrating birds. I vividly remember how creepy they looked and sounded. Their loud collective cries freaked me out and I couldn't wait to get back in the car. Needless to say, I never made it to the end of Alfred Hitchcock's disturbing movie, *The Birds!*

Over the years, my aversion to flying creatures continued to be fed by my utter disdain for the thousands of pigeons invading the streets and parks of London.

In January 2019 though, I found myself developing a soft spot for birds when a flock of Vulturine guineafowls happily crossed the dust track in front of our Jeep in the middle of the

Masai Mara. They looked so bizarre, with this odd combination of a tiny vulture head and a disproportionately big body shaped like a football. What makes them so stunning though is their plumage: Their necks and breasts are covered with thin long white and grey feathers layered over a striking bright cobalt-blue undercoat. The rest of their big oblong body is dressed in white polka dots on dark grey feathers.

We had already stopped so many times that morning to eagerly observe and take pictures of giraffes and elephants that I quickly grabbed my phone and poked my head outside of the moving jeep to capture the slow-moving flock (besides, I didn't want to show too much enthusiasm for birds).

"Oh yeah, my mom LOVES birds!" exclaimed my daughter, knowing full well that I DO NOT. Tim, our jeep driver, with his usual understated kind demeanour spent the whole rest of the day stopping at EVERY sighting of birds and even made little detours to find more birds for me to take pictures of! My daughter was trying to contain herself from bursting in laughter. She has the wittiest sense of humour that one just can't get enough of. Always coming up with the funniest comments or observations that one can't but wonder how she does it.

Back in London after this once-in-a-lifetime trip exploring Kenya, worrying news about Covid-19 were spreading fast. The contagion gathered so much momentum that just over a month later we all found ourselves in lockdown to contain the spread. No one had predicted that it would be such a somber year for so many. Mourning for millions of families, near-total isolation for millions of elderly people, desolation and depression. Businesses closing their doors, people losing their jobs, our social circles deflated. On the other hand, a myriad of stories of generosity and kindness lightened up our world and gave us renewed hope.

My respite came in the form of our one hour outdoors daily exercise allowance. Not an ounce of my body enjoys jogging so I set out to walk in St James's Park every day after lunch. The weather being unusually glorious for pretty much the whole of the lockdown, I'd sit on a bench by the pond halfway through my walk to soak in a bit of sun. All around the pond are displayed clear signs NOT to feed birds and yet, there's always someone carrying a huge bag of breadcrumbs, enthusiastically scattering them all over the place and attracting tons of bloody pigeons. I had to keep my cool despite a pressing urge to ask them if the signs were not obvious enough. After a few days, I decided to just let it go. I was coming here to contemplate the beautiful surroundings so letting my blood boil would defy the purpose.

As I sat there, on the same bench, day after day, the time often coincided with my daughter calling me. She could obviously hear all of the birds and ducks in the background and would tease me, calling me a 'bird lady'. I'm afraid this nickname may follow me for a long time!

One day though would be different from all the others. Like a déjà-vu scene, I was sitting, watching the same man throwing breadcrumbs left and right by the pond. Watching the same birds, ducks, ferocious swans and geese, fight for the last pieces on the pavement in front of me. From a distance I could see the park police van slowly approaching, making its afternoon social distancing spot-check round. The flock had gradually dispersed as the vehicle progressed. I was simply observing and suddenly, right before my eyes, I saw its front left wheel run over a large black bird's lobed foot, crushing it.

The bird had obviously not seen the van coming. No other birds had hurried him away. It must have been in such agony yet, all alone, it painstakingly hopped on one foot and made its way back into the pond. It didn't even occur to me at the time to alert the park rangers. I stood and looked for it but it seemed like it had vanished amidst the hundreds of other feathered creatures.

Tears came pouring down my cheeks. They were the saltiest ever. Filled with pain, sadness and guilt. They brought me straight back to when I was little, watching my younger sister get hit by a car we had not seen coming. A distracted driver had ignored a stop sign and sped around the corner towards us. I had not hurried her away in time. In a flash, it happened. In an instant, she laid there in the middle of the road. I can only remember one horrific scene: My sister bouncing off the pavement on her head, and a car. That's the beginning and the end of what I recall. Melted together in one horrific instant. Nothing else.

That black coot's suffering would become my blessing, little did it know. It made me face what I never had the courage to let go of: Guilt. Even though I had no control over that car driver's actions, I still felt like I could have grabbed my sister in time. Above all, being the eldest, I should have known better but to cross in the middle of a street even if there were no car in sight...or so I thought.

Weeks passed and it became clear that I needed to ask for my sister's forgiveness. I went back, sat on the same bench, called her and told her everything. I apologised for having crossed the street ahead of her, for not having protected her, for not remembering anything thereafter. For her suffering. She lovingly forgave me. She actually never held any resentment nor did she know of the guilty baggage I held onto for years.

Asking for Forgiveness

Forgiveness is not merely an act you choose to perform towards someone who's done you wrong. If you have been carrying something you need to be forgiven for, a most transformative gesture is to ask to be forgiven. Only you know what it is and the instances will vary widely throughout your life. It can be for something you deliberately do or didn't do. In most instances, expressing remorse, taking responsibility, making amends and asking 'can you ever forgive me' will sow seeds of peace. In your heart and the other's. If the person decides not to forgive you, you've still shown that you are willing to change. In their own time, they may be more open to forgiving. Regardless of whether you receive forgiveness or not, your conscience will be clear, and you will raise your own bar for extending forgiveness to others. Forgiveness is cleansing and transforming for all involved.

We cannot live in harmony within ourselves when we carry a guilty burden.

Do you carry guilt for which you need to be forgiven? Who would you want to ask forgiveness to?

Forgiving Someone Else

Do you carry resentment or anger or hate towards someone you need to forgive?

We all do.

In a way, forgiving someone who's done you wrong is such a challenge in that, most often, the offender doesn't acknowledge nor want to acknowledge the pain they have caused you, or they don't care, and in some instances, they haven't even realised they've hurt you. They might also be fully aware and don't give a damn. Not only can you feel deep resentment, but often time, anger builds on top of it because you know they don't care and you'd wish for retribution. And you replay the scenario in your head over and over again!

We may think that by not forgiving someone we are somehow getting back at them, but in reality, it damages us. Our anger and hatred cause our hearts to become disfigured, hindering our ability to love and find peace within ourselves.

Think of how all those feelings add weight to the massively heavy load you are now carrying on your shoulders? Think about what it does to you? The pain you inflict on your body against your own will? You and your body become all out of balance, completely misaligned.

We all know that we are called to forgive and of course, the scriptures and many other religious texts address the subject. Often times though, despite knowing that we are called to forgive, and why we are called to forgive, we just don't know how. It's like you try and it comes right back at you.

Could we think of letting go first and then forgive? Or, just letting go? Is that even enough?

It is well known that forgiveness benefits the one who forgives and that unforgiveness is like a poison building up inside us.

In trying to grapple with the actual act of forgiveness towards a few people who have hurt me, here's what I found helpful and I'm hoping that you can take something away from it, if you also struggle. Bear in mind that this is by no means a method which trivialises some extreme circumstances you may have gone through, nor the act of absolute divine forgiveness extended to all of us.

A Big Duffle Bag

If you carry a heavy bag on one shoulder, you will eventually feel the strain. Walking in itself will become difficult, you'll be lopsided. You may even have built stronger shoulder muscles on one side to bear the weight. Over time, whether you shift the heavy bag onto another shoulder or keep it on the same side, the pain will become part of what your body expects, impeding it from functioning optimally. Perhaps even leading to injuries. You will try quick fixes and they will at best temporarily compensate for the pain.

The same goes with unforgiveness, it totally disrupts your balance. It affects you in ways that you will come to subconsciously expect. Living with it becomes a normal part of your existence. It weaves into all of your being. It lives in you and through you. You may not consciously notice the imbalance it created because you've been carrying it for so long that it became a familiar thing.

You can let go of that familiar ill.

Your unforgiveness burden is not carried by the one who's done you wrong. It is the bag you carry on your own shoulder. If you wait until they offload that heavy bag from you, you will wait a long time! The heavy bag is on YOUR shoulder not theirs. You are carrying it, not them. Most likely, they don't even know nor care that you are carrying it.

Seeing it in this way has helped me tremendously with letting go and in finding a step forward towards the ultimate act of forgiveness which is to extend love to the person who's done you wrong. In many cases, I decided to let go of that heavy bag as a form of detachment and to regain my own balance. Can letting go be a first step in our journey towards forgiving? Can letting go of that heavy bag, leaving it by the road help us detach from it and even give us the ability in the future to walk past it and see it in a different light? After having had the time to reset ourselves straight? Would we be willing then to actually empty its contents?

Forgiveness goes beyond 'letting go' and it implies absoluteness. Choosing to extend mercy and love to the one who offended you.

A Prison Inside Your Heart

My deepest hurt, one that sent my body and soul in a state of shock, came with the news that the person I loved profoundly wanted to go his own way. We had spent thirty years together, sharing all of life's wonders. It felt like I'd been robbed of life itself. The past and the future collided, leaving a massive black hole in my heart, sucking all of life's joys, memories and dreams. The only way to live at peace was to go beyond letting go to fully forgiving. Forgiving myself in love, forgiving him, in love. But, how? I couldn't just let go because despite the hurt, I knew that walking past the heavy bag I'd leave by the road side, I would still feel the pain. I needed to do more than unloading the heavy bag. Going beyond that unloading to saying, "I forgive you," and meaning it full circle. I needed something I could relate to. A 'how' to go along God's commandment. A way.

One day, I stumbled upon a video in which a lady brilliantly put into words just what I needed to do. I don't like methods per se but I was open to listening. It was beautifully profound yet simple, and I could totally relate to how she framed it. Too simple perhaps? I will let you ponder...

Here it goes:

Think of a prison, set inside your heart. See the person you need to forgive chained to prison bars inside your heart. Stay with the image while absorbing how it feels. You can do this once or repeat over a few days if you need to. Then, take a key, open the heavy metal door, and let him/her go. No just go, but go in loving peace. For your sake. For their sake.

If it is yourself being held behind your own prison bars, do the same. With compassion and love. Forgiving oneself may sound elusive or evoke sentiments of being undeserving. Wishing to feel better about oneself may also seem like a moral transgression, even if we firmly believe that others deserve compassion. You are just as deserving. Self-forgiveness is just as important. Remember this.

Who wants to be the host of a heavy prison in their heart and let unforgiveness stain their soul? No one.

My heart no longer hosts a prison. I've forgiven myself from my own mistakes. I've disassociated the hurt from my love for him. That love will never go away and as such, it can surpass anything. The form has changed, and such is life.

As the months went by and the sun had warmed the earth, I moved from my bench to lying on the soft grass below majestic trees, marvelling at the vastness of the sky and the huge canopy of mature twirly branches above me. Birds everywhere. The city was immersed in quietness, you could actually hear them sing. What were they teaching me now? What can they teach all of us? To rise above. Rise above the bitterness. And when we do, it looks so calm from up there. Gracefulness, calmness, wisdom.

Final Thoughts

Many say that forgiveness isn't about the other person but about our own emotional freedom. Yes, emotional freedom is essential for our wellbeing yet making forgiveness about us AND the other person is the ultimate gateway to complete peace.

Receiving the gift of forgiveness is an absolute blessing. Forgiving is a noble sacrifice.

We all have been forgiven at some point for our mistakes... why shouldn't we also forgive?

Let go, forgive, love. It's the key.

This chapter is dedicated to my beautiful sister. A woman with a great sense of love, dedication and endless courage.

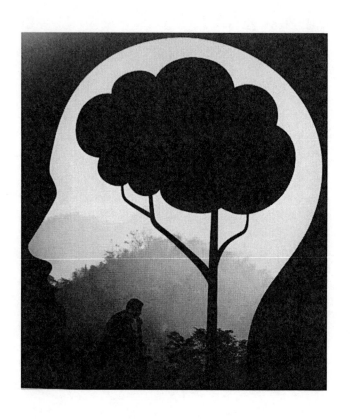

Chapter 7
Deep Minding
There Is No Secret

What's at the core of our power? The power which drives our lives, the power with which we can achieve our purpose, the power we have to choose, heal, love, create.

We are bombarded daily with news of how big tech enterprises are dominating our lives and how they have become empowered by each and every one of our personal and collective profiles. At the essence of this propulsion towards conquering increasingly greater frontiers is their ultra-savvy use of artificial intelligence. Not until I was exposed to this concept (and had to learn about it, not by choice, but by necessity!) did it become somewhat of a fascination which I'm hoping will also trigger in you some rethinking about how to shape what drives your own power.

Let's first take a quick look at artificial intelligence and what it means in simple terms. The engine driving AI's growing power is machine learning. Machine learning algorithms use statistics to find patterns in massive amounts of data. This data encompasses a lot of things; numbers, words, images, clicks, and the list goes on. Machine learning is the process that powers many of the services we use today: Netflix, YouTube, Google, Instagram, Facebook and voice assistants like Siri and Alexa, to name but a few.

Each platform collects as much data about you as possible: The genres you enjoy watching most, links you are clicking on, posts you are reacting to and uses machine learning to make highly educated guesses about what you might want next.

This reality goes even further. Deep learning, for the sake of simplicity, is like machine learning on steroids. It employs algorithms to process data and mimic the human thought process. It uses layers upon layers of algorithms, to understand human speech or visually recognise objects, for example. The data, similar to the chemicals passing through our brain neurons, is transported via synapses, travelling from one layer to another, providing input for the next layer of information. It goes so deep that it can generate the most precise patterns. Not only will it find patterns in your behaviour, but it will also predict patterns and influence you into adopting new ones.

Algorithms pretty much rule the world by organising and making sense of data for us, although, something even more powerful runs your world if you tend to it and know its ways: Your mind. The core power over your thoughts and actions. If our brains initially inspired deep learning, deep learning could inspire us to explore more of the majesty of our mind and all of its layers.

One of the most profound discoveries of my late forties (better late than never!) was that our thoughts have the tremendous ability to shape our lives, for good or for bad. That every action was the result of a thought. That life was not 'happening to me' but that I had a greater say in how I wanted it to unfold.

Never had I paid particular attention to how my reality was defined until I hit a brick wall, experienced huge stresses and had to do something about it. My reality did not serve me well at all, nor did it serve my purpose in life.

More than two thousand years ago, even Jesus spoke of the renewal of our mind, changing the way we think in order to create a better life for ourselves and a life that honours God.

"Do not conform to the pattern of this world, but be transformed by the renewing of your mind. Then you will be able to test and approve what God's will is—his good, pleasing and perfect will"
Romans 12:2, NIV

The Mind

"That which feels, wills, and thinks; the intellect."
etymonline.com/word/mind

Our mind is our power machine. It is more than just our intellect and powerhouse of thoughts, but through our mind, we feel and will. We will to grow, love, give, etc.

Your thoughts, memories, feelings, are the codes which make up the program in your mind. Over time, they add up, intertwine, and get engrained into the many layers of a program which runs your life. If your program is not generating the results you desire, could it be because the patterns you have created are faulty? Remember, algorithms operate on huge sets of data. If you have allowed, over and over again, 'self-deprecating' and 'worst-case scenario' kind of thoughts to filter in, they are now fully embedded in your programming. Your program runs on that data, just like machine learning algorithms learn from the data presented to them. The more data, the more accurate the end results.

After spending a lot of time examining the kind of thoughts I was entertaining, examining my habits and beliefs, it all started to make so much sense. Reshaping my thoughts was something I had to do for my health and also for the way I interacted with others.

By choosing to explore the content of the life-program you've been running on, you can break free from the unconscious reality and circumstances you actually don't want to find yourself in. A program is a program and it can be changed. The effort required is greater than simply letting the same program run but nevertheless, it is totally feasible and exciting.

Let's Explore

Everything in the world begins and happens as a result of the power of thoughts. Think about it, everything around you was once just a thought. Every bridge you see was once an architect's plan. The world itself is said to have started as a thought from God. Look around you and observe how everything material started as an idea. Thoughts are therefore inherently creative. This applies to both positive and negative thoughts. Take a second look, beyond the materialistic world, and see how most of your reality is a mirror to your thoughts and beliefs. Take these examples: 'I'm just not good enough to apply for this job', 'I'm always too tired to exercise', 'he's better than me', 'there must be something wrong about me'. Those assumptions lead to feelings of discouragement and will likely cause someone to put in less effort. That lack of effort will only reinforce their beliefs.

Or, maybe you accepted, and still accept, what someone told you when you were growing up, 'you're not so good at this', 'if you are not the best, you will never make it'. If you accepted those thoughts, even though they were wrong, they have shaped your life. Can you see how they contribute to produce a version of yourself that is lacking in confidence and self-worth?

The most vital exercise we can do as leaders of our lives is to examine, program, re-program, and also weed out the viruses that often seep through the filter of our minds (think of manipulative advertisements, social media falsehoods and filters, etc.). If we don't, the culture and environment will do it for us and allowing this to happen will cut us off from our own greatness and happiness.

> *"Be careful how you think; your life is shaped by your thoughts."*
> *Proverbs 4:23 GNT*

There Is No Secret

Consider this: In drawing a conclusion about ourselves, we are likely to look for evidence that reinforces our self-beliefs and discount anything that runs to the contrary. Our reservoir of information has been filling up for years so we draw from the same old pool of data.

Take a close look at the labels you've placed on yourself. Have you declared yourself inferior or too old, too young, not experienced enough, not attractive enough, not educated enough, too thin, too fat, a failure, or doomed? Now, observe your personal circumstances. Can you see them as proofs of those labels?

If someone develops the belief that he's a failure, for example, he will view each mistake as proof that he's not good enough. When he does succeed at something, he'll accredit it to luck or see it as a one-time off. His mind will focus on seeing the negative occurrences in his life; becoming attuned to them, amplifying their significance, and being oblivious to the positive things that are happening.

You don't have to allow those beliefs to continue dictating your life and keeping you tied. Just because you think something, doesn't make it true. What you are experiencing is familiar, but think about it honestly, would you rather be familiar with a sub-par life or explore possibilities of a new reality?

How about THE secret to manifesting your new reality, attracting what you desire?

There is actually NO secret.

Rather, you need to switch your self-talk to: 'you are good at this', 'you are healthy', 'you attract good people', 'you are blessed with happy relationships', etc. What happens then? Your mind programming absorbs those thoughts and the feelings they create. You become attuned to them and your focus shifts to seeing the good in your life. You naturally engage in relationships that are fruitful, you naturally make healthy life choices, you naturally find ways to improve your knowledge, etc. If you start thinking that you are rich, health wise and financially, the choices you make and the information you consume will be in line with your new philosophy of life. You will naturally gravitate towards seeing the good, making good choices and exploring the best options. Those choices will add up and create the new patterns you have chosen for your life.

The purpose is not to manifest a mansion within a week nor about fooling ourselves or satisfying our egos but rather, getting satisfaction from living a fulfilling life, with integrity. That in itself will bring about more positive changes, in and around you, than you can imagine. You will also see the not-so-good circumstances (as there will be some) as one-offs, and no longer as the main drivers of your life.

> *"Until you make the unconscious conscious, it will direct your life and you will call it fate."*
> *Carl G. Jung, Swiss psychiatrist*

About Making Changes

You must clearly identify who you really want to be. What kind of life are you aiming for? If you fail to make a conscious decision you will naturally bend towards the undesirable. All humans do. Sort of like an unattended field or garden that grows wildly with anything that blows by. Anything left uncared for will ultimately degrade. If you want to grow in a way that leads to positive changes, you are going to have to do so intentionally, and put in the effort.

You can garden your mind in many ways.

How Do We Make All of This Work for Us?

By doing some 'deep minding'.

Catching the ill-serving codes we let in. Being mindful and aware of those thoughts when they happen.

Removing old codes and detaching from their feelings.

Adopting new codes and associating them with new feelings.

In exploring the many meanings of 'minding', we will make our way to adopting lasting positive changes that will weave into the deep layers of our minds.

Here are some to ponder and use as checkpoints in your own 'deep minding' journey:

Minding as in to pay attention to

You can decide how you want to live by examining your self-talk and the thoughts playing in your mind. Are they negative or positive? Do they make you happy? Do they bring you down? Are they serving you or not?

Are they thoughts about your past you are beating yourself up with? We often hear that the past is past and we can't do anything about it. The past exists in our minds and may have left unwanted scars in our present. What we can do now is to be grateful that it brought us to this new awareness and we get to press reset. In paying attention, especially through meditation, we can see those scars, process them, let them go. Freeing space to experience our new reality.

Minding as in to be aware

Mind what's happening around you. How do you react? How do you engage? What are you letting in? How does it make you feel?

Our thoughts are fed by the conversations we have, songs we hear, news we watch, books we read, interactions we have, advertisements we see, and the list goes on. Be aware. Our conscious mind impresses our subconscious mind. The subconscious mind expresses all that is impressed upon it. It accepts as true the ideas which the conscious mind feels to be true. Since our subconscious mind transcends reason, it contemplates feelings as facts. Be aware.

Minding as in to tend to

Your thoughts are a force, and an energy that you can direct to work for you. You must tend to your thoughts in the knowing that they are inherently creative. What would you like them to create? How can they enrich your life? You must also tend to your self-talk. Self-talk is a powerful tool and it's your best friend. It can also be your enemy. Make it your best friend always. You live with self-talk 24/7. What would your best friend tell you? And how? Remember that.

Minding as in to be careful about

Mind your own business. When you focus on someone else's business, you basically give your own power away. Think about it...you are wasting it. Spend that time and energy on building yourself. You will be much better served.

Mind about dwelling on imperfections and wrongs about others or yourself. It impresses your subconscious mind with those limitations. Rather, ask yourself what you can do to positively deal with them.

Mind about idealising something or someone you've missed out on (who knows if it would have been good anyways?) and make sure you focus your mind on what's real, healthy and worthy.

Minding as in to make certain that

Make certain that you take time to expose your mind to sources of information that build knowledge and are positively transformative. That you create circumstances that trigger your best thoughts.

Engage yourself in learning more about the power of your mind. The science is ever evolving and it is an exciting field to explore. Look into what one of my favourite contemporary great minds, Dr Joe Dispenza, has to say on how we can rewire our brains and recondition our bodies to make lasting changes. He is an international lecturer, researcher, corporate consultant, author, and educator and he is driven by the conviction that each of us has the potential for greatness and unlimited abilities.

> *"If you focus on the known, you get the known. If you focus on the unknown, you create a possibility."*
> *Joe Dispenza, Becoming Supernatural: How Common People Are Doing the Uncommon*

Minding as in to be cautious about

Mind the traps.

We can get so accustomed to the negative emotions some thoughts generate that they become all but too familiar and, in a way, we find comfort in them. This unconscious trap we fall into is the victimisation of our circumstances. It's a very powerful and deceiving trap. We often turn a blind eye on it since it can be the hardest thing to admit to ourselves as it takes a direct hit on our pride. How can it be that we dwell on living with a victim mentality? Consciously or unconsciously, it happens. Why?

Firstly though, let's not conflate being the victim of a crime or a serious offense with the concept of victimisation of our circumstances.

We are addressing the idea that we all feel sorry for ourselves from time to time or powerless in the face of a monumental challenge.

In harnessing a victim mentality, you will see your entire life through a refractory lens, meaning that things happen 'to' you, they hit right back at you. It means viewing most things in life as beyond your control and expecting sympathy. Sympathy makes us feel loved. It fills a need for attention.

The not-so-easy aspect to admit to ourselves is that a victim mentality can be a means to sheer away from taking responsibility for our lives. In believing you lack the power, you unconsciously justify to yourself that you don't have to take action or you unconsciously justify the frustrations in your life.

Familiarity thus becomes appealing, even if you're not conscious about it. Don't get stuck with a situation or a thought and say, "That's just who I am or that's just how my life is." Since a victim mentality is a learned behaviour, you can indeed 'unlearn' it. By catching yourself when it happens, you can choose to transform your life by entertaining new thoughts and creating new habits.

As you become aware of this trap, you will notice that beyond random bad occurrences, many things in life happen because of the choices you make and that you have the power to choose differently. You will also recognise that when misfortune happens, it will have nothing to do with being deserving or not because you will have reconstructed the mind program you operate by. You will rationally and clearly distinguish the events for what they are.

Minding as in to be careful of not letting your thoughts define you but rather, define your thoughts.

One other very important aspect I would like to touch upon is that our thoughts do not define us. This is a concept I just could not get my head around. How is it that, when I am the one thinking and observing some pretty dreadful thoughts in my mind, those thoughts are not me? They must be a representation of me? Everything I read on the subject says that 'you are not your thoughts' but not really why exactly that is. I mean, I can actually produce, at will, some rather awful thoughts so, how is it that I am not my thoughts? After all, I am the one generating them! The best answer I found came during a massage therapy session while chatting to the therapist (yes, I am one of those who always tries not to chat away and just relax but ends up engaging in hour-long conversations!). Speaking of the bad thoughts I catch myself entertaining and why they are not me, she said: "Those awful thoughts you just thought about came from the *you* that you were five minutes ago when you thought them. You are already a new you, having recognised them and choosing now that you don't want to keep entertaining those thoughts." I was obviously bothered by the origin of bad thoughts but in the grand scheme of things, there is a constant stream of thoughts that actually just flows in and out of our mind without making much of an impression. It is what we choose to obsess over or focus our attention on that we can question and act upon. Thoughts will come back but we will have a different background upon which to process them (especially the bad ones!). It's in the context of our awareness that we can choose if and how to process them.

Renew your mind, as you go along. You will renew yourself and continue to grow, as you go along.

Minding as in to keep in mind

Do keep in mind why you are doing this. You are developing your self-awareness and cultivating your life.

Do keep in mind that every time you blame someone or your circumstances, you are giving away your power to be the change you want to see. You are indirectly feeding that someone's ego or your circumstances.

Do keep in mind that the more effort you allocate to your own growth, the less control you will need to exert to find inner peace. We can say that we are all pretty much control freaks, in one way or another! Many of us often micromanage things or others because we are not comfortable dealing with imponderables or not being in the driver's seat. Instead, we ought to shift our practice to exercising more control around the discipline we engage in.

Do keep in mind the remarkable power of your feelings. Our thoughts don't exist in isolation. We think and feel, all the time. When you think of something, it is most likely making you feel a certain way inside. Going back to our conversation about discipline, when you are thinking of yours, reinforce it by imagining how it would make you feel. Happy, relieved, proud, energised, calm or excited. How do you want to feel on the path to achieving your goal?

Final Thoughts

Just as 'deep learning' predicts patterns of and influences future behaviour, 'deep minding' will become the key to creating the new patterns that will drive your future thoughts and actions.

Shallow doesn't stick. We must let our new patterns sink in.

When you deeply renew your mind and align it with what is good in the world, you will experience so much more peace and harmony in all aspects of your life.

Addressing yourself as the leader of your own life, you will no longer say, "I'm not good enough" but rather, "This is not good enough."

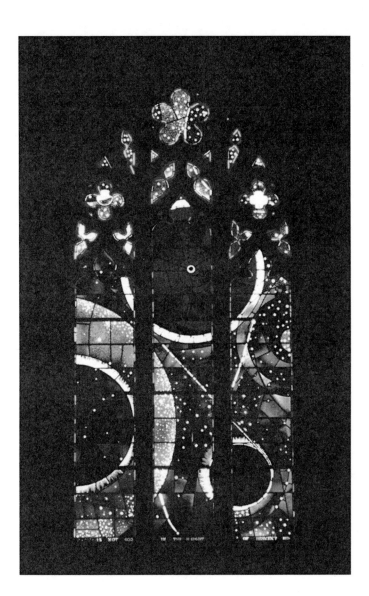

Chapter 8
The Power of Prayer
Even If You Don't Know
How to Pray

If you ask any Washington D.C. resident where they were on the afternoon of August 23, 2011, they will remember, vividly.

On August 23, 2011, a magnitude 5.8 earthquake hit Mineral, Virginia, about 90 miles southwest of Washington D.C. The temblor was the strongest east of the Mississippi since 1944, and was felt by more people than any other quake in U.S. history, reaching 12 states. It shook the nation's capital so strongly it cracked the Washington Monument and caused upwards of thirty million dollars in damage to the National Cathedral.

The earthquake's seismic energy shot up through the cathedral's highest elements 'like the tip of a whip' shaking its intricately carved pinnacles and slender spires, sending finials and angels plummeting, causing heavy stones to rotate dramatically and flying buttresses to crack. "It was like a punch to the gut," said Joe Alonso (head stonemason), describing the shock and disbelief he felt as he surveyed the damage for the first time from the top of the 300-foot central tower. (*smithsonianmag.com*)

When the earthquake hit D.C., the seismic waves reached the highest part of the city, which is the hill the cathedral sits on. The waves travelled up to the highest part of the building, severely damaging three of the tower's four pinnacles, cracking dozens of flying buttresses, jarring columns out of place and knocking a 350-pound hunk of carved stone off the northwest tower and onto the ground outside the main visitors' entrance. Miraculously, no one was hurt.

Washington National Cathedral is one of the most distinctive landmarks of the D.C. skyline, with its Gothic towers, its elaborate stained-glass windows and, for the past ten years, its scaffolding. The building is majestic and the magnificence of its interiors, breathtaking. The cathedral is adorned by two hundred stained glass windows, bathing the inside in the loveliest pastel light you can imagine. One of the most unique, the Space Window, holds a treasure. Shining at the centre of a deep red sphere is a round piece of white glass containing a sliver of moon rock. The lunar chip is approximately 3.6 billion years old and contains a previously unknown mineral: Pyroxferroite. 'Piece 230 of Apollo 11 rock no. 10057' is the only moon rock ever given by Nasa to a nongovernmental institution. The sample was presented by Neil Armstrong and fellow Apollo 11 astronauts Buzz Aldrin and Michael Collins as 'a fragment of creation, from beyond the Earth' – to the Cathedral on July 21, 1974, to commemorate the fifth anniversary of their first steps on the moon. (cathedral.org)

Standing below the window, appreciating its beauty and reflecting on its spiritual and scientific connections to the mystery of the cosmos, is quite a moving experience. Every Wednesday at the end of the school day, I got to drive my daughter to her one-on-one flute lessons, held at National Cathedral School, which shares the same grounds as the Cathedral.

Its magnetism drew me in every week, at the same time, during the hour I had while she was at her lesson. The moment I walked in, I felt calm and blessed. I'd quietly sit in a pew, soaking in a little extra piece of life, absorbing the beauty all around me. The timing was absolutely perfect. An Evensong was sung by the school choir and included the reading of Scripture, followed by a short sermon. It might just be the most beautiful soulful hour in all of D.C. For those of you who are not familiar with a choral Evensong, it is an abbreviated church service traditionally held every day as the sun goes down, marking the passing of another day in faith and allowing for contemplation.

The Cathedral is designated as 'a house of prayer for all', no exceptions. Not only does it pursue interfaith dialogue and collaboration, particularly among the three Abrahamic faiths, but it also seeks to promote reconciliation among all faiths and compassion in our world.

Its designation as 'a house of prayer for all' is quite significant. Prayer is humanity's common healing practice. It is understood by all, of all faiths, and of no faith. One doesn't need to be religious to pray. And, ironically, one doesn't really know how to pray in order to pray.

Think about it for an instant. Its reach is beyond measure and borders. We offer prayers for nations and strangers who are going through tragedies. For friends and loved ones needing moral support or encouragement. We also offer prayers for good luck wishes and success. Prayers of thanks for an achievement or news to celebrate. Prayers are pure and bound us in hope.

Prayer in Solitude

Months had passed since my daughter's first music lesson and the Cathedral had become my weekly hour-long refuge. Had it been preparing me for something? I believe so. A severe hip injury left me walking with the aid of crutches for weeks. The pain was so intense that having to stop dancing for months meant it was really, really, bad. I was shattered. Perhaps that's how a musician would feel if his instrument was taken away from him. Prayers for healing came from friends and family but I needed to do my part, too. Do you often wait until you are hit with a bad situation to pray? I did.

Weekly physiotherapy sessions did not seem to be helping much at all and I couldn't even fathom ever being able to get back on the dance floor. My ultimate recourse was to devote myself to prayer, there was no other way. I'd think that God would prefer us to be more diligent with our prayers but, still, he's a gracious and utterly patient God.

I made my way to another Evensong with a specific objective in mind: To pray for miracle healing and believing that Jesus had healed me. Basically, fully trusting and committing to this promise of his:

"Therefore, I tell you, whatever you ask for in prayer, believe that you have received it, and it will be yours."
Mark 11:24 NIV.

It was almost like I was putting Jesus to the test so I felt a bit bad. Or, was it Jesus challenging me?

To my utter amazement, both the Bible passage and short sermon, were literally meant for me. It could not have been clearer, there was not even an ounce of doubt. I cannot claim that God 'speaks' to me, although that day, he clearly did. And it was certainly not a coincidence. Have you ever read accounts of people saying that God speaks to them? Have you, like me, ever wondered how exactly? I had asked a friend who had claimed several times to have heard God's voice to describe specifically how it manifested and I always got nebulous answers.

I absolutely did not hear any voice coming from heaven but God was addressing me directly by way of the scripture being read and the sermon delivered on that day.

Did I exit the Cathedral sprinting down the nave? No. Had I been miraculously healed? Yes. How did I know? I just knew to trust that my prayer had been answered and the Evensong of that day was a gift for me. I walked out rejoicing and thanking Jesus profusely. I walked out in the absolute knowing that I was healed and the manifestation of this healing was already on its way. Full healing was already in progress. I believed it. There is one other very important thing I needed to do: Thank those who had prayed for me and let them know that Jesus had healed me. Not only in his mercy and grace does God heal but he heals so that in turn we can give him the glory he deserves, and inspire others to pray.

Prayer is talking to God and waiting on his presence, not just asking for things. And just as it is with a friend, you cultivate a relationship and you do not turn up only when you need something. Prayer is an attitude of your spirit and heart that reaches out to God. Prayer is not a formula nor a string of empty words. If there is a void in your heart and your voice is silent and you want to pray, that desire will be known to God. That desire brings you closer to seek after Him, in your own way. It opens doors to exploring resources that will guide you and that you can relate to.

Had God been preparing me for months? Showing up and seeking him? His timing is certainly not ours. Sometimes this waiting will seem like an eternity.

"God knows our thoughts," Pastor Jack continued, "but He responds to our prayers. We have to come to a place of realising that prayer is a privilege that is always ours, but the power in prayer is always His. Without God, we can't do it. Without us, God won't do it." *(faithgateway.com)*

Prayer is an opportunity to centre us, pause, thank, pour out our heart, and invite God, the divine, to participate in the affairs of our life.

Prayer is also a remarkably touching experience for humanity and a most powerful agent in transforming the heart. It moves us to take action.

Prayer in Community

Two years later, at a time when my husband was struck with desperation and panic, I needed to go back to the Cathedral and pray with all the might I could muster. My husband was on the very edge of not making it through the week. It was the saddest and most terrifying moment I had experienced in my married life. I had even written, clearly with a sense of urgency, to our dear pastor and his wife: "I thought I was going to lose him. He started crying and grabbed his head saying that huge anxiety and physical pressure go into his head and that he was breaking down, not knowing what's happening with him (despite medical tests that were all fine) and said he'd need to be locked up on a psychiatric ward soon. It lasted more than an hour. I don't know what to do anymore. I'm trying to be strong, pray for him, comfort him but it's getting worse and worse. Thanks for your prayers, lots of love."

That night, as he went to bed, I sat by him, softly reading Bible passages. I can't remember which ones. I just didn't have words of my own. Perhaps God was guiding me, it's all a bit of a blur. I read until he was able to calm down.

I begged him the next day to meet me at the National Cathedral for the service and we'd stay for a while longer to pray for him. I thought, if Jesus healed me there, he could heal my husband too. Whoever attends the service is kindly invited to the praying chapel – known as the War Memorial Chapel – afterwards if they so wish. Knowing that the pastor who leads prayers in this intimate chapel always asks the attendees if someone needs to be prayed for, I stood up and went to the front asking permission to read a note out loud. Between having delivered presentations to a large company's executive committee and reading an emotionally filled plea for help to complete strangers in a church, the latter took a monumental amount of courage. I was looking at them and at my husband with tears rolling down my cheeks. What happened next was an outpouring of love from the people there who bowed their heads in prayer and one by one came to put a gentle hand on his shoulder. Some were clearly visitors, perhaps even from a different faith and others would have been locals. It didn't matter because the common act of prayer, whichever prayer they prayed and however they prayed, was what united us.

Just like I had walked out of the National Cathedral a couple of years earlier, I believed that my husband had been healed as well. I trusted God. Along with the power of prayers from many, the love from his family and friends, and the care from a specialist, he made it through. Just as with my own experience, there was no instantaneous healing but deep down in the calmness of his heart, below the extreme agitation and anxiety, must have rested the knowing that he was safe. That it was going to be okay.

Prayers sustain us. Prayers are a gift that can never be forgotten nor lost. There is no shame or weakness attached to offering a prayer, whether you are a believer or a non-believer. On the contrary, it delivers on a heightened sense of selflessness and compassion.

What are your own experiences with having been prayed for or having offered the gift of a prayer?

Prayers Know No Boundaries, From One Faith to Another

For years, whilst living on the outskirts of Washington D.C., we have had the immense blessing of having a wonderful lady come by, twice a month, to help with cleaning the house. When I first met her, I thought she was in her forties...not a wrinkle. Imagine a tall woman, quite robust, dressed with colourful layers and a little on the timid side. She could have very well been a bodyguard. She would actually become our family's soul guard.

Despite excruciating pain in her feet, Isa (who was in fact a grandmother in her late sixties and not timid at all!) always showed up. It initially took me a bit by surprise when she asked if she could take the time to pray Dhuhr. I was humbled by her small request and touched that she felt at ease to pray in our house. She made praying a priority between busy tasks.

Years had already passed and we looked forward to her coming by. She brought laughter and love, told me tales of her life in Gambia and hilarious stories about her cheeky granddaughter.

The very first time we had to leave her the keys, as we were going on a holiday, I sat down with her to go over a short list of instructions on operating various appliances, and which lights to turn on or off during our absence.

I could sense some uneasiness. Isa was illiterate. My heart sank. She shared her story and her big dream of one day being able to fill out a customs form on an airplane on her own, without being stared at for asking for help. Without feeling inferior. Without living in constant fear of being judged for not having the basic knowledge to read or write whilst navigating this crazy world.

There is one thing that Isa could read very well though: Our hearts. She'd check on us and pray for us, at times of hardship and at times of celebration. Never did she miss a birthday or a holiday, sending us a recorded message, always ending with 'I'm praying for you'.

After she was done with her work, we started English lessons in our kitchen. The joy in her eyes. She was a bit distracted, which was actually quite funny, and always so keen to show off her progress with reading and writing short words. Her binders slowly filled with pages of new vocabulary and illustrations. Months went by and she could write and read simple sentences. We were so proud of her.

Sadly, our stay in the USA had to come to an end and it was time to say goodbye. A goodbye filled with tears and hope, too. Isa was family and always will be. To this day, we still chat and she even replies, on her own, to text messages. It is a long road ahead before she is able to fill out a customs form on her own but I know she can.

Our prayers will bind us together forever. Abaraka, Isa.

"Our job in prayer is simply to seek God, sit before Him, pour out our hearts to Him, and then trust Him. Give him all that we are, whatever we are facing. Because the ultimate triumph is all His, over the whole of this life, over the whole of eternity."
Rev. Jamie Haith, St George's Church, Bloomsbury

Final Thoughts

Take a moment to recall the impact prayer has had in your life, as a receiver and a giver. Pray in silence as you walk by someone who looks sad. Pray with thanks for a friend's achievement. Pray for your family's good health.

If prayer feels or seems dauting, you can find a gold mine of inspiration online and in books to guide you.

God is in the height of heaven for everyone.

Prayer is key to reaching anyone's heart.

I dedicate this chapter to my then husband, who always stood by me in prayer and love, and who still does. Now from afar.

Parts of the proceeds will be offered as a gift to Isa to pursue English lessons.

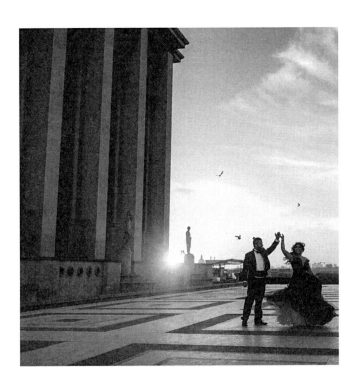

Chapter 9
Your Body and Its Temple

His name was Michael Jackson. My first love. Bordering obsession. I had a poster of him, sporting his iconic red leather jacket, at the back of my bedroom door and I'd kiss him goodnight before going to bed. Yes, I really did. And when MTV released his first music video, *Thriller,* in December 1983, it was like nothing else existed in my world.

There had been nothing like it. A full 13-minute video of sheer magic and excitement. Dance moves like no other. It reignited my dreams of becoming a dancer. Instead of studying, I'd sneak to the basement of our house where the TV was and watch the video on repeat for hours to learn the moves. My aim was to nail the whole dance choreography.

My parents though were less than thrilled when I told them I wanted to become a dancer, the likes of those who appeared on music videos. Bless them, with the best of intentions, they cleverly steered me towards pursuing a business career. That path took me to where I'm at today and I wouldn't have it any other way!

Dreams rarely die though. They shouldn't. We ought to let them live or take a slightly different form if we are at a different stage in our life.

About six years ago, I found myself completely mesmerised, sitting in a spectacular ballroom in Central London. I had travelled from the USA to participate in a dance competition, and also watch the top professional Latin dancers in the world compete. I was there to cheer on an American couple I knew but my attention quickly shifted towards two stunning dancers from London

She had immediately caught my eyes. A beautiful young woman with an exotic look. There was something special about her. Dancing in a gorgeous black dress decorated with bright yellow, orange and red flowers, she moved with such femininity and passion. You could see it through her eyes all the way to the tips of her fingers. He commanded the floor, oozing charisma with his magnetic presence and chiseled figure. He let her shine and together, they produced something truly unique and magical to watch.

The ways in which the universe works are often mindboggling. They are now my teachers and have both already enriched my world beyond the dance studio walls. As UK professional Latin champions, Marika and Gunnar embody what they teach: fullness, fluidity, high standards and uniqueness. Those principles have helped me move and express more of myself on the dance floor but also in life. I would like to share them with you, as I believe they provide a distinctive and compelling backdrop for how we can best carry ourselves as we progress through life.

Our soul and body take us from one place to the next. How can we best equip them both to do so?

Building Grace

Who will preach in your temple?

A graceful temple stands firm, with elegance. It houses and embodies its soul. It is built and maintained over time. And, to stand the many tests of time, it is supported by a team of masters in their fields. Our temple, body and soul, needs the same as we continue to build, maintain and fortify it. In doing so, many will have the opportunity at some point in their lives to turn to a coach, mentor, teacher or therapist to learn a new skill, perfect an existing one, or for therapy or advice. You ought to choose wisely who you let inside your temple, who will come 'preach', and who will truly be invested in you. Letting in the ones whose motivations and intentions are sincere, and whose values align with yours. Some may be popular but remember that popularity doesn't necessarily make a temple greater. And just like eating unhealthy food over time, the energy inside your temple will be off until you find those who genuinely support your growth. Those who meet you where your needs need to be met.

Only after having to leave a teacher whom I thought was unparalleled did I understand that he hadn't been the best fit for me. I'd never bothered thinking about it, or I knew but didn't want to admit it to myself for fear of having to make a change. Can you relate to that?

Are you confident about who is preaching in your temple? About their principles? Are they the best fit for you now? Choose to build a temple that will evolve with time and with grace.

What's behind what you see?

In dancing, as with most things in life, including our relationships, superficiality is a disguise. It is bound to make something crumble at some point and when something crumbles, it hurts. Emotionally or physically.

Superficiality revels in masking deceptiveness, shallowness, a shaky foundation, or a lack of self-confidence, for example. Think of a fake façade from a movie set. Deceptively real. But what's really behind it? What is it trying to represent?

Superficiality blinds us even though we can spot it even before the lights come on. It blinds us to what's real and meaningful. We even scroll through it every day.

When it comes to who preaches in your temple, follow your intuition and your trained eye. Look for authenticity and integrity. Your temple ought to stand true and strong.

Live life on and between the beats

I remember hearing Jay Shetty say during an interview that the biggest part of learning something is actually 'unlearning'.

Years of focusing on an end product, making something look good, or wanting to win is not so easy to 'unlearn'.

I was taught to be quick on my feet (which is not a bad thing!) and dance to the beat of the music (which is also not a bad thing!). But what happens in between the beats? The music still plays and that space invites us to explore more of it. How to unlearn steps and learn how to express our body?

Life is lived on and in between the beats. Just like in dancing.

It is a principle I'm constantly being reminded of during my lessons. Our legs dance to the beat and our body dances to the melody, with fullness and fluidity. Finding how one movement produces another sounds pretty simple yet it's one of the most challenging and beautiful aspects of dancing. It requires strength, flexibility, balance, and great awareness. The same goes with life. To go from square one to your next destination requires a whole lot of skills and applying learning from accumulated experiences. The more you develop your skills, the more you will fully explore what lies between each step of the way. Between each step, you make beautiful discoveries and notice more opportunities. They will become treasured experiences. Be conscious and find enjoyment in the space that leads you to your next step.

Is there an area in your life where you would also need to 'unlearn' something? Where what you do just seems like a means to an end? Are your skills sufficient to take you to the next level?

Our development and willingness to explore new ways of moving from one level to the next are often limited by our comfort zone and our lack of awareness.

On your journey, choose a friend, mentor and/or coach who leads you to fully explore your potential between point A and B. Who challenges your ways. Who puts in the real efforts, just as you do.

Reflect on who is preaching in your temple. Rarely do we go through this exercise, don't we? Gage them before engaging with them.

What and how are they contributing to your life, on and in between the beats?

How have you been evolving under their wings?

Evolving physically, and as a whole

Just as with any physical activity, dancing teaches us to keep our core muscles 'in' or 'engaged'. In doing so, our foundation is more solid and less prone to injury.

It teaches us that our core (or centre) is like a bridge connecting our legs and upper body. If we don't engage our core muscles, the energy between the top half of our body and legs is interrupted. We can think of it just like an open bascule bridge, where nothing can flow from one side to the other.

It also teaches us to take our core one level up. Not only keeping our core muscles 'in' but consciously lifting them up. At first, I thought that it didn't make any sense. Why would I want to feel lifted up from the ground as I moved? Wouldn't I slip or fall? All but the contrary. In elevating our physical core as we move, which also elongates our spine, it provides more space for our muscles to freely move. It frees up space to take deeper breaths. It also, counterintuitively, grounds us even more firmly to the ground.

Just as a simple exercise, you can stand and feel the floor with both feet, core muscles tucked in. Now, lift your centre. Can you feel your contact with the floor increase?

These physical notions, learned through dancing, can teach us something about how we carry ourselves through life.

An Elevated Life-core

By keeping a strong core of values within you, by standing firm onto them and by elevating your standards, you create more room in your life to experience growth. You expand the space within you for what truly matters. You feel more grounded. Being a grounded person means that you have a strong connection with who you are which in turns brings emotional stability. You stand balanced no matter what is going on around you. You live your life with intent and you are in tune with your thoughts and emotions. You stand with conviction within your own body. Harmony flows throughout your body.

Of course, we can dance without engaging and lifting our core muscles. We can live without standing tall and firm. But why limit ourselves? We have the tools to expand our bodies and minds.

With an increasingly grounded poise and a strong elevated core, you are creating more space within you for what truly matters. To freely experience and create. To actively expand your range of possibilities. In expanding this range, you will seek opportunities to fulfil them. Transform your desires into words. Interact with people who have achieved what is a currently a dream of yours. Take your first step.

"Dancing is like life. The lessons of one are the lessons of the other."
Savion Glover.

Walk to the moon, on repeat

I now know the drill! When my lesson starts, I must do laps around the floor doing 'rumba' walks in slow motion. Apparently, the very best Latin dancers never ever stop practicing rumba walks. Or at the very least, not until they've performed enough of them to cover the distance to reach the moon. That would roughly be half a billion steps or fifteen years of walking non-stop!

Acceleration then becomes a real temptation. How often do we want to move ahead, move on, fast? Faster? It's far less of a thrill having to endlessly repeat a skill, break it down further, add something new to what you already know, and then, repeat the cycle all over again.

Rather than using seemingly satisfying and precipitous strategies, a wise coach will tie your progress to bite-size and sustained achievements so that you feel increasingly confident about yourself and your potential.

They will want you to fully grasp the skill you are learning or fully explore as many tools as possible to navigate the challenge you are confronted with. They will constantly search for ways to best tailor their message to your needs.

They will make repetition a discipline you will come to appreciate and seek. It teaches your body and/or brain to become one with what you are doing. As it becomes one with you, you will move, work or think with precise intention, and at a greater speed if and when need be. Speed becomes an asset rather than a means to cut corners or avoid putting in the effort or the time.

What we are in the process of learning is bound to suck. It certainly did for me, and still does but the benefits have somehow extended to all of the other dances. True progress with any part of your body or mind positively impacts the rest of you. It wonderfully permeates through many other aspects of your life.

Keep at what you are developing, with intention, repetition and patience, and enjoy it. Your body and mind will welcome the effort, and your ever-improving abilities will become a part of you and how you move. Your body and mind will reward you. From one slow motion to another slow motion or from slow motion to warp speed, as long as it's moving, keep at it.

"Hustle Beats Talent When Talent Doesn't Hustle."
Gary Ryan Blair.

And just when you think you're getting good,

'I got it!' That feeling when we nail something. It's actually a really good thing we get it. It keeps us motivated, especially after weeks and months of learning and practicing. It also comes with a fine print: "Be aware, complacency is bound to set in."

Just as I am finally able to dance some challenging parts of my choreographies at a relatively decent level, they start to go on a gliding trajectory. Gliding downwards, that is! My teacher immediately notices: "Let's do it again, and again and again! Make this moment, any moment important. All. The. Time."

You might have already seen this diagram from Bruce Lee:

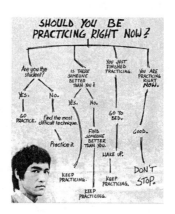

Firstly, the fun way with which he presents his message always makes me smile. His look is stamped in my head! Secondly, I love to use this analogy for how we ought to view our progress with any skill we are working on. This has taught me the importance of noticing what I need to constantly revisit and polish in my own life. It is also a great reminder of the importance of making every moment important.

Can you think of an area in your own life where complacency may have set in? If so, how can you address it to redress it? Imprint Bruce Lee's look in your mind!

Grow beyond your cocoon

A great teacher/coach will be enthusiastic about your attempts at trying and will always find ways for you to push your limits.

Outside of our comfort zone, we grow, find amazing things about ourselves, and we develop more confidence. Learning to explore beyond what feels or looks familiar makes us more malleable. Self-consciousness transforms into self-confidence. The first many times I was asked to improvise a short solo piece of dancing before my actual choreography starts, I wanted to crawl under the floorboards! That push outside of my cocoon became part of the learning experience. It was like that annoying piece of a puzzle you want to give up on finding but really need in order to continue the section you are working on. That really tough piece to find which looks like all the others but has a tiny yet defining detail that makes it unique. When you do find it and it fits, it beautifully completes the picture, and ultimately the puzzle. What you find, do and learn outside of your comfort zone completes you. It brings out your uniqueness. It's the necessary needed piece.

Outside of our comfort zone, we also unconsciously develop new brain-body connections. The more we build them, the more they will get activated. The more open we become to doing something that would have otherwise made us feel like we just couldn't. The more we build new healthy connections, the fuller we live, and the more confident we become.

Is there something you ought to be challenged with in your life to continue to progress? At work? In a sport you practice? In your studies? Do you know which piece of the puzzle you ought to find?

Choose someone who values uniqueness

There are trends in all disciplines and in pretty much everything in life. My dance teachers have chosen to stick to their own path. They believe in the value of investing in what makes them unique as opposed to investing in becoming like others on the competition floor. It is a risk that solid individuals are willing to take. They have embraced they own trend. They keep their focus on what they are doing rather than being engulfed in what everyone else is doing, concentrating their efforts as opposed to diluting them. They will win some and lose some but, in the end, they will have achieved greatness.

As Gunnar's puts it so clearly: "Embracing your uniqueness is being true to yourself and accepting yourself for who you are. There is no magic bullet, your goal should just be to be a better version of yourself even if it means taking baby steps day by day. And if you find yourself unhappy with what you see or feel, then the responsibility is with you rather than others. At the end of the day, the ultimate reward will be that you listened to your own heart and lived with your instinct instead of relying on other people's opinion."

A great coach/teacher will nurture this uniqueness in you. They will guide you while letting you be you. They will value you. They will teach you in a way that you will become a better version of yourself so that you can continue to grow and shine. Marika puts a great emphasis on this as she teaches: "I guide my students but also give them the freedom to explore their movement because only then will it be genuine, authentic, and theirs."

Whether it feels daunting or unfamiliar, whether it comes easily or takes a lot of time, they will understand your challenge as they will have experienced it for themselves. You will achieve your own greatness rather than your version of someone else's. If you don't have such a person in your life to guide you at the moment, you can nurture this notion of uniqueness for yourself. In being aware of why it matters. In embracing your flaws and gradually changing the way you do things. Within your own field. Ultimately you want to value being you, filtering in what is constructive and motivational, and using it wisely to shape who you are. Filtering out unproductive or shallow opinions. Making your temple unique, one of a kind!

How do you value your uniqueness? How do you manifest it in your life? Or are you swallowed up in the bodies of those you envy, of those you nourish from?

The ultimate dance lesson: How do we connect with one another

How many times have I been told not to push or pull my teacher/partner while dancing? With time and experience, it

125

became clear that the more strength, flexibility and coordination I developed in my own body, the less I needed to rely on my partner to keep my balance or to move from an especially challenging step to another. With those improved skills comes a greater ability to express my own movements. And, ironically, the more I can do on my own, the better we can move together.

This connection between two individuals in dancing mirrors the interdependence found at the core of any healthy relationship. Dancing with a partner teaches us so many lessons, enough to fill the pages of a book on its own. On this particular aspect though, one can draw a parallel with how we move in our own lives, as an individual and in a partnership, and how we can better understand the value of interdependence over dependence.

While my dance partner leads me, I strive to keep and manage my own balance and I don't disturb his, and vice versa. We both allow one another to freely express ourselves. We are both able to feed off the other's energy to move and follow. Of course, it is a learning journey and I still needlessly push and pull him in various places, yet those become markers for where I need to continue to train my body.

From these few principles, we can draw valuable lessons for how we connect in any of our close relationships.

That is, aiming to maintain a solid sense of self within any relationship dynamic while recognising and valuing the importance of the bond you share. Identifying problems along the way, just like in dancing, as markers for where one or both individuals need to adjust and improve. Pushing and pulling never leads to anything harmonious.

Lastly, you will often see a dancer completely leaning on another, thus creating spectacular movements or captivating moments of stillness. Before any of this can happen, those dancers have trained extensively to be able to maintain their own balance.

Do you have a good sense of your own balance in your relationships? Is your self-worth dependent on the other person? Can you stand on your own?

Are you needlessly pushing, or pulling?

Cultivate an awareness of what you stand for on your own, what you stand for together, and what you need to work on.

Final Thoughts

By investing in your body's overall health, in keeping your temple strong, you will feel grounded and better prepared to face life's challenges.

Give the key to your temple to coaches, mentors, therapists, friends, partners who enrich your life.

*If you notice an intruder,
you will know best what you ought to do.*

*If you ever dreamed of dancing, it is never too late to start!
It's never too late for any of your dreams.*

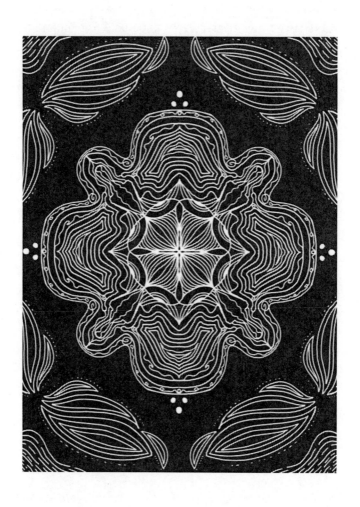

Chapter 10
The Theory of Everything
In Search of Equanimity

You have most likely been asked this question at a dinner party: "If you could invite a guest from the past, present or future, who would it be, and why?" Tough pick!

My intention was to wrap up this book with a special guest who embodies the many subjects we've discussed throughout. I thought long and hard and finally chose someone of impeccable virtue and character from whom we could learn, and whose humanness we could connect with. A special guest who transcends the past, present and future. You will meet him soon and he will share his keys to living with equanimity.

Do you have a favourite bedside table book? Taking it with you in your carry-on wherever you go? Showing signs of time throughout like it has been lived in? Highlights, ink underlines, sticky notes poking out from the pages, chunks of pages no longer attached to the spine. Folded corners, grease stains?

One of a few, now discoloured and looking as if I wrestled with it, found itself following me for over ten years. *A Briefer History of Time,* by Leonard Mlodinow and the late Stephen

Hawking. It was published as a more accessible and updated version of his initial worldwide bestseller, *A Brief History of Time*, addressing the ever-fascinating subjects of the nature of space and time, the role of God in creation, and the history and future of the universe. Where did the universe come from and where is it going? Did it have a beginning? What was before then? What is the nature of time? Will it ever come to an end? Why does the universe go to all the bother of existing? Will we ever have a theory of everything?

Although, *A Briefer History of Time*, is literally somewhat briefer than its predecessor, and purely technical notions were replaced with broader concepts, the bottom line is that I lost the plot less than a halfway through! I'd tackle it every year with renewed ambition thinking that the information would sink in and that I'd be able to hold a somewhat intelligent conversation about black holes, singularities, string theory, particle velocities and curved space, but alas.

Despite the growing frustration and the book having now found itself in a box packed for our next move, I had to give myself another chance to finally 'get it'. At the announcement of UK's first full Covid-19 pandemic lockdown, I signed up for an online beginners course in astrophysics and supplemented my learning with Brian Greene's World Science Festival videos on YouTube. It was so much fun, by lesson eight, I thought I would nail it.

By month number three, it felt like Brian Greene had become a close friend. I'd even started dreaming about him, black holes, quantum realities, extra dimensions, entanglement and the mysteries of space. I attended a couple of his live World Science Festival lectures where he was taking and answering viewers' questions in real time. I know that there are no stupid questions but the ones I was dying to ask would have forced him to contain a massive rolling of the eyes and a pretty much guaranteed sigh of exasperation. So, I didn't dare.

By month four, all my hopes were crushed. Unless I'd marry a Brian Greene, that was it for my astrophysics dreams. Despite not wanting to give up, I nevertheless had to come to the evidence…

Not all was lost though. I found an intriguing takeaway from Hawking's book and Greene's videos, which offers an elegant proposition for our human lives: the search for a *unified theory of everything*.

Many physicists are tirelessly concentrating their efforts to find a single, all-encompassing theory that describes the entire universe. A 'Theory of Everything' that would unify Einstein's general relativity – the gravity-based science of the very large – and quantum mechanics, the science of the very small, subatomic particles and forces.

You might be asking yourself what the significance would be for humankind to even bother with finding a theory of everything to describe our universe? I surely did!

This is Steven Hawking's answer:

"If we do discover a complete theory, it should in time be understandable in broad principle by everyone, not just a few scientists. Then we shall all, philosophers, scientists, and just ordinary people, be able to take part in the discussion of the question of why it is that we and the universe exist. If we find an answer to that, it would be the ultimate triumph of human reason – for then we would know the mind of God."

Honestly, I don't think we will ever know the mind of God even we find a complete theory of the universe, but it certainly will bring humankind closer to its quest!

Could WE also live by a 'unified theory of everything'? More specifically a unified theory of life? One which, in our life, unifies the science of the infinitely small with the science of the very large. Bringing together the invisible force within us and the universal force which connects us all.

Let's Examine...

What is the invisible force within us?

Beyond our powerful minds, well into the core depth of every single cell in our bodies, is divine intelligence. Loving, creative, powerful divine intelligence.

If the divine power or intelligence created the first elements at the origin of the universe, and we are made from those same elements, we each hold a parcel of the divine. Infinitely small, yet beyond anything we can imagine. The fact that all matter is composed of the very same substance, says a lot about our interconnectedness and the single source of life.

God. Intelligence. The divine. I am aware that not all readers are Christians, although most people believe that we originated from a greater, unique, divine and powerful source. Looking into the great religious, spiritual, and wisdom traditions, we find the precept that life's ultimate truth, its ultimate treasure, lies within us. Jesus, in saying that the kingdom of God is within us, gave voice to a teaching that is universal and timeless.

This powerful divine intelligence is also the infinite force which connects us all. Everything is interconnected, made from the same source. Through our thoughts, emotions, beliefs and actions, our words and our relationships, we are responsible in unifying the infinitely small yet powerful intelligence at the core of our being with the infinitely vast power which connects us all. Developing as individuals and participating to the common good. Collaborating to the common good.

How Can We Unify Those Two Principles in Our Lives?

With equanimity.

I would like to suggest that living with equanimity is our *human being theory of everything* and it binds together all of the elements we have discussed throughout this book.

In my humble opinion, Buddhism offers the most elegant description and expression of equanimity:

"Neither a thought nor an emotion, it is rather the steady conscious realisation of reality's transience. It is the ground for wisdom and freedom and the protector of compassion and love. While some may think of equanimity as dry neutrality or cool aloofness, mature equanimity produces a radiance and warmth of being."

Ref.: Gil Fronsdal (2004-05-29). 'Equanimity'.
Insight Meditation Centre. Retrieved 2009-07-21.

In and of itself, the word equanimity provides us with a blueprint for what lies at its core. From the Latin: *Aequus* (even) and *animus* (mind), the word means 'balanced mind'. Only from a balanced mind can we become aware and accepting of reality's transience. Only from a balanced state of mind can prosper wisdom, freedom, compassion, and love. Our state of mind imprints our actions.

I have learned the hard way, one too many times, that there has to be harmony between having a balanced mind and living accordingly to get a taste for equanimity. Our actions are a mirror to what our minds look like. A good look at our actions is a good indicator of the state of our minds. Examining, learning, and getting better at what we do and say. If time is a healer, time is also a teacher, and a gift. Held and felt in the 'now', it's a present. Rolled out into the future, it is a gift that gives us a continuous stream of possibilities. Possibilities to balance our minds and cultivate our actions.

How Can We Live with Equanimity?

In unifying the invisible force within us and which connects us all with a constant search for and display of wisdom, freedom, compassion and love in all we do.

By accepting life's transience. The universe speaks to us through its constantly changing nature. Letting go of our resistance to change has to be our answer to let the energy of life flow. Knowing that everything in our lives is impermanent (the good and the bad), we no longer grasp at certain conditions, people, or objects, hoping to hang onto them. No longer are we at the source of our own suffering because of a reliance on being attached to something in order to feel secure.

Circumstances change, we change, people come and go. We ought to let go when the time comes. We ought to also learn to accept how other things are going to go and be at peace with it.

Let Me Introduce You to My Dinner Guest

A humble man who was constantly searching for equanimity amidst his struggles. Constantly striving to show love and compassion. His acceptance of the ephemeral and changing nature of life fed much of his wisdom. His stoic discipline of mind gave him the freedom to experience life with harmony. He also expressed a deep reverence for the divine in his life and at the source of life.

Perhaps I have watched the movie Gladiators one too many times! I can't but picture him elegantly dressed in a sumptuous toga, riding on a majestic horse. A piercing look through which all of his life's challenges are melted into one singularity. A skin bearing the fine prints through which he navigated life. A wise, resolute and charming smile. And, a tear, carved on his cheek, from the gripping decision he had to make at the end of life in letting his sadistic son become his successor.

Marcus Aurelius (121–180 AD) was the last of the 'five good [Roman] emperors', known to have ruled Rome with authority, humanity, and competence. He ascended as emperor upon the death of Antonius, his adopted father. He was ostensibly a man of great intelligence, peace, composure and compassion, yet he spent most of his reign at war. At the time of his death, he would have been one of the most powerful people on earth and he proved himself deserving of the power he held. Under him, the empire was guided by virtue, wisdom and love.

Referring to a friend/general who betrayed him, Marcus would 'forgive a man who has wronged one, to remain a friend to one who has transgressed friendship, to continue faithful to one who has broken faith'.

He left us an extraordinary gift in the form of a most unique literary manual: His private notes to himself – *Meditations*. The twelve books (similar to chapters) of *Meditations* were a source for his own guidance and self-improvement. It is said that it is unlikely he ever intended the writings to be published. Through reading *Meditations,* we are left wanting to become a better person and to put all of its wisdom together in our own unified theory to living a fulfilling life.

Marcus Aurelius' book also exposes many of the problems we deal with today and the same problems we will be grappling with tomorrow. Concepts trending nowadays can almost find their roots, word for word, in Marcus' *Meditations* from nearly two thousand years ago.

"When force of circumstance upsets your equanimity, lose no time in recovering your self-control, and do not remain out of tune longer than you can help. Habitual recurrence to the harmony will increase your mastery of it."
Meditations, Marcus Aurelius.

Condensing such a treasure chest of reflective and practical wisdom proved to be a nearly impossible task but one I thought would solidify all of what we have discussed throughout this book. Here is my selection of Marcus' observations and guidance that can best illuminate our paths towards our search for equanimity.

On Relinquishing the Present Moment:

"When the longest- and the shortest-lived of us come to die, their loss is precisely equal. For the sole thing of which any man can be deprived is the present; since this is all he owns, and nobody can lose what is not his."

"Each of us lives only now, this brief instant. The rest has been lived already, or is impossible to see."

Book III

On Wisdom and Integrity:

"Not to let others hold you back. To locate goodness in thinking and doing the right thing, and to limit your desires to that."

Book V

"Nowhere you can go is more peaceful than your own soul. Renew yourself."

Book IV

"Because most of what we say and do is not essential. If you eliminate it, you have more time, more tranquillity. Ask yourself at every moment, 'Is this necessary?'"

Book IV

"What humans experience is part of human experience."

Book VIII

On Having a Balanced Mind:

"The things you think about determine the quality of your mind. Your soul takes on the colour of your thoughts."

Book V

"Stop allowing your mind to be a slave, to be jerked about by selfish impulses, to kick against fate and the present, and to mistrust the future."

Book II

"Your ability to control your thoughts – treat it with respect. It's all that protects your mind from false perceptions – false to your nature, and that of all rational beings. It's what makes thoughtfulness possible, and affection for other people, and submission to the divine."

Book III

On Self-compassion:

"Don't be ashamed to need help. Like a soldier storming a wall, you have a mission to accomplish. And if you've been wounded and you need a comrade to pick you up? So what?"

Book VII

On One's Responsibility to Others and Empathy:

"Care for other human beings. Follow God."

Book VII

"Practice really hearing what people say. Do your best to get inside their minds."

Book VI

"For as these were made to perform a particular function, and, by performing it according to their own constitution, gain in full what is due to them, so likewise, a human being is formed by nature to benefit others, and, when he has performed some benevolent action or accomplished anything else that contributes to the common good, he has done what he was constituted for, and has what is properly his."

Book IX

On Always Moving Forward:

"Stop drifting."

Book III

"Dig deep, the water goodness is down there. And as long as you keep digging, it will keep bubbling up."

Book VII

"External things are not the problem. It's your assessment of them. Which you can erase right now. If the problem is something in your own character, who's stopping you from setting your mind straight? And if it's that you're not doing something you think you should be, why not just do it? But there are insuperable obstacles. Then it's not a problem. The cause of your inaction lies outside you. But how can I go on living with that undone? Then depart, with a good conscience, as if you'd done it, embracing the obstacles too."

Book VIII

On Living in the Present:

"Even if you're going to live three thousand years, or ten times that, remember: You cannot lose another life than the one you're living now, or live another one than the one you're losing. The present is the same for everyone."

Book II

"Everyone gets one life. Yours is almost used up, and instead of treating yourself with respect, you have entrusted your own happiness to the souls of others."

Book II

On Discipline and Freedom:

"Do external things distract you? Then make time for yourself to learn something worthwhile, stop letting yourself be pulled in all directions. But make sure you guard against the other kind of confusion. People who labour all their lives but have no purpose to direct every thought and impulse toward are wasting their time – even when hard at work."

Book II

"Concentrate every minute...on doing what's in front of you with precise and genuine seriousness, tenderly, willingly and with justice. And concentrate on freeing yourself from all other distractions. Yes, you can – if you do everything as if it were the last thing you were doing in your life, and stop being aimless, stop letting your emotions override what your mind tells you, stop being hypocritical, self-centred, irritable."

Book II

"Don't waste the rest of your time here worrying about other people – unless it affects the common good. It will keep you from doing anything useful. You'll be too preoccupied with what so-and-so is doing, and why, and what they're saying and what they're thinking, and what they're up to, and all the other things that throw you off and keep focusing on your own mind."

Book III

On Interconnectedness:

"Keep reminding yourself of the way things are connected, of their relatedness. All things are implicated in one another and in sympathy with each other. This event is the consequence of some other one. Things push and pull on each other, and breathe together, and are one."

Book VI

"Everything is interwoven, and the web is holy; none of its parts are unconnected. They are composed harmoniously, and together they compose the world."

Book VII

"When you need encouragement, think of the qualities the people around you have; this one's energy, that one's modesty, another's generosity, and so on. Nothing is as encouraging as when the virtues are visibly embodied in the people around us, when we are practically showered with them."

Book VI

"People exist for the sake of one another; teach them, then, or bear with them."

Book VIII

How do you see yourself cultivating equanimity on a day-to-day basis?

Final Thoughts

With a balanced mind comes groundedness in your thoughts and actions.

This groundedness and harmony lead to a greater appreciation for life's transience, and greater space to let wisdom, freedom, love and compassion grow within you.

"Mature equanimity produces a radiance and warmth of being."

Don't we all long for this radiance? A radiance shining inwards and outwards, bringing warmth and joy to our soul and to those do around us.
Could that be the ultimate key?

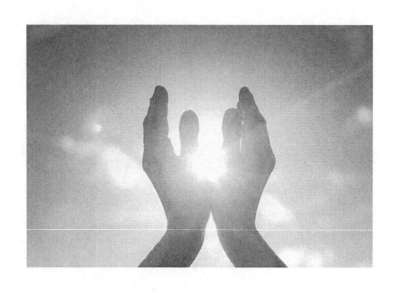

Chapter 11
Reminders and Compass-Setters

We all have a collection of lessons we've discovered and learned from over the years. Through time, experience, people, challenges, adversity, and good fortune. I love reading about people's take on life as it enriches my own ever-growing philosophy on our journey together here on earth.

I would like to share with you, in no particular order, the lessons that have become my compass-setters. This compass has to be reset regularly as I can be all over the place even during one day. I am hoping that some will find themselves relevant and helpful to you, too.

Say I love you, I miss you, you mean so much to me, I thank you, to someone every day.

Call your parents as often as you can. They love you. Who knows if they will still be around tomorrow.

Thank God every day. That your child is alive. For you family. That you woke up. For your loving pet. For your awesome body. For his protection and grace even when you have no clue how he's working behind the scenes. Have you ever wondered about that?

Say, 'I am aware' a few times every day. I am aware that I am breathing. I am aware of the beautiful blue sky, of the slow-moving clouds. I am aware that this too shall pass. I am aware that I am loved.

Smell the grass, wet or freshly cut. The leaves, flowers. Connect in any way you can with nature. Even just a conscious glance at a tree, admiring its beauty.

Before you go out the door, leave your home like you'd want someone to find it.

Laugh. If nothing makes you laugh today, find laughter by watching a comedy clip or call a friend who makes you laugh. Read silly funny posts. Watch one of those hilarious pet videos. Laugh at yourself. Smile at a stranger as you walk by. Smile softly as you close your eyes.

Downshift. Reduce the speed. Walk slower. I used to walk as fast as possible to kill two birds with one stone; to save time and burn as many calories as possible so I wouldn't have to do a workout! I ended up wasting time, not appreciating what was in front of me, and building up useless stress.

Stretch your body and mind. Your body: You are not flexible? One millimetre more every day. Watch where that takes you. Your mind: Learn something new every day. One word. One chapter, one podcast, one article. Switch hands when you brush your teeth. Developing new connections in your brain, regenerating and renewing yourself constantly. You will become more malleable as a person, also developing new connections with those around you.

Eat chocolate, taste it, enjoy it. One square. Two squares. Delight in that irresistible cupcake, in that dollop of cream over sweet strawberries. One life. Good balance.

Work with what you have as opposed to fight for what you lost. Your hair is going grey, wrinkles are redefining your face? Use your smile to glow, rather than unnaturally fight just to be left without looking like yourself.

Put that plastic in the recycling bin. A big effort? It's not an effort, rather, our responsibility. Sharing one world together. Better yet, don't buy plastic. Cardboard tampons, ladies.

Do one act of kindness and shut up about it. In giving or doing, it doesn't matter. Something beautiful doesn't need praise, it's inherently beautiful.

Fill out that annoying survey to compliment someone for their good service. It may lead to a recognition or a promotion and help their family.

Go away. Travel. Get lost. Make memories. Engage with other cultures. If you have children, take them with you. They will learn beyond what the classroom will ever teach them.

Rest your body and mind. Meditate, sit or close your eyes on the train or while you sip your coffee. Listen to music. It doesn't have to be long.

Privacy is sexy. Integrity is sexy. Uniqueness is sexy. Be sexy then.

We never know what's around the corner. It can be good or not so good but everything is ever-changing. Move and change with it. The world will go by without us if we stay chained to circumstances. Staying permanent through life's impermanence keeps us stuck.

Detach from idealising something or someone. You don't even know what is really lurking under their façade. The one minute you spend idealising someone or something is one less minute to better yourself. Keep this power within to build yourself and grow.

Stay away from drama. It sucks your energy. It's a net negative.

If you think you are right, pause and ask yourself: "What if I'm wrong?" Be in a position to be intrigued by another's views or opinions and to see the world as it is, as opposed to how you think it should be. Be in a position to defend your ideas when warranted.

You can push a door to open possibilities. If it doesn't open after a few attempts, leave. There is a good reason it can't be forced open. A '*no*' here can take you to a better '*yes*' somewhere else.

There is always a solution. A way through, a way around or a way in another direction.

Final Thought

"This life is for loving, sharing, learning, smiling, caring, forgiving, laughing, hugging, helping, dancing, wondering, healing, and even more loving. I choose to live life this way. I want to live my life in such a way that when I get out of bed in the morning, the devil says, 'Aw shit, he's up!'"

Unapologetically You: Reflections on Life and the Human Experience
Steve Maraboli